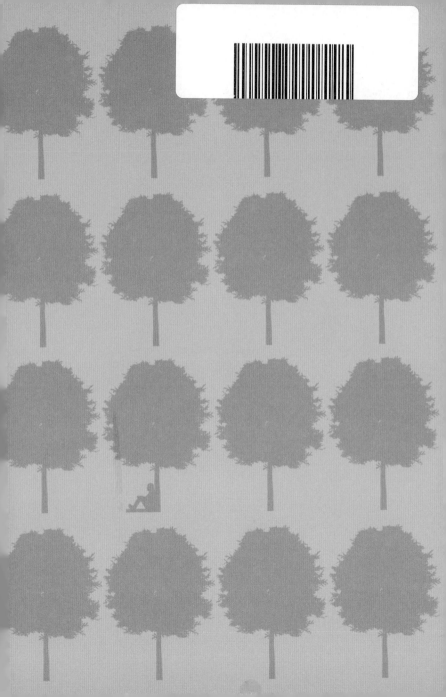

The Sweetness of a Simple Life

DIANA BERESFORD-KROEGER

THE SWEETNESS
OF A
SIMPLE LIFE

Random House Canada

PUBLISHED BY RANDOM HOUSE CANADA

Copyright © 2013 Diana Beresford-Kroeger

www.randomhouse.ca

Random House Canada and colophon are registered trademarks.

LIBRARY AND ARCHIVES CANADA CATALOGUING IN PUBLICATION

Beresford-Kroeger, Diana
    The sweetness of a simple life / Diana Beresford-Kroeger.

Includes bibliographical references and index.
Also issued in electronic format.

ISBN 978-0-345-81295-7

    1. Conduct of life. 2. Simplicity. 3. Home economics. 4. Traditional medicine. I. Title.

BJ1595.B47 2013   646.7   C2013-900754-7

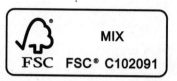

Cover and text design by CS Richardson
Cover, end paper, and title page images: musicman and gst, both Shutterstock.com

Printed and bound in the United States of America

10 9 8 7 6 5 4 3 2 1

This book is dedicated to Money Bags,

Douglas Alexander Hart,

who wanted and got the skin off my custard.

Contents

Life has become complicated, and this complica-
tion is not necessary. Everybody needs time
for themselves. The daily swirl of constant activity
that we subject ourselves to steals our time. Time
is our most precious possession. To give somebody
your time is to give him or her part of that precious
thing. You can only offer such a gift by simplifying
your life so you have time for yourself and more,
again, to give away.

It is only through living simply that we will be
able to navigate the future. Adopting simplicity
will streamline your life, your health and your mind.
Your children will benefit and even the people who
work with and around you will reap rich rewards in
empathy and more human contact. Marriages benefit
from simplicity; love feeds us all, just love, simple
and supreme. Our lives should be filled with time for

it. Your children are waiting for it. Even your pet is waiting for that extra little pat, today.

I have written this book to help you reset the clock. Each essay is built on science, a practice I have spent my life pursuing. In some ways I believe that science has stolen the innocence out of modern life, but without it we would not have all the improvements of everyday living, ease of transport and communication. We are all stuck in that forward momentum of science, but with each essay—on the health of your body, the food you choose to eat, your hearth and household, your backyard and garden and the world all around you—I am offering you a new wellspring of simplicity to use to your advantage. Each such choice and change helps simplify and strengthen the larger environment we all share.

Let me tell you a little about myself (the rest you will just have to guess from what I do not say). I was orphaned in Ireland as a young child, an aristocratic mongrel. In my mother's family were the ancient kings of Munster, Ireland. My father was a scion of the great Beresford family, which includes earls and lords in both Ireland and England. The judge was afraid to plant such a child in a Magdalene laundry orphanage and asked me into his chambers for my advice. Opting to stay with relatives, I went to live with a bachelor uncle, my mother's brother, Patrick O'Donoghue, in Cork. He was a feted athlete, a scholar, and owned an immense library of first-edition books in Irish and English from all over the world. I dived into those books and some of them, with my uncle's handwritten notes on philosophy, religion, theatre and poetry, sit breathing Canadian air in my own library now.

In the summers other relatives on my mother's side, all in their eighties, plucked me from Cork and brought me to the countryside of Bantry Bay and Glengarriff. They were Irish speakers and kept the Celtic traditions alive. Over three summers, they drilled me in Celtic culture and the ancient knowledge of the Druids, and tried to prepare me to survive in what they called "the new world." They told me, "You will be the last voice of the ancient Celtic world. There will be no more after you." In the fall and winter and spring, I went after education like a starving dog goes after a bone. I was a Beresford child from a prominent Protestant family in a Catholic girls' private school. The nuns brought in the heavy artillery for me from the local university. According to my uncle's wishes, I was as free as a bird to study. Every single night we took turns reading either physics, philosophy or poetry to one another by the fire of turf and coal. It was like we grew up together, in some way. He was advanced for his time because he really believed that women should be educated.

So I went to university, first in Cork, and studied for a double first in medical biochemistry and classical botany. In my final year I took over from my professor of botany who became ill, and taught the year. Then I did a master's in plant hormones and frost resistance. I went to the United States on a fellowship and studied for my doctorate in molecular biology with a minor in radionuclear chemistry. In Canada, I continued my research and I completed a diploma in experimental surgery. Most of my work in Canada has centred on hemodilution, open-heart surgery and the biochemical work in this area. I refused a professorship in medicine because I preferred to travel in my own line of thinking, which is looking at holistic systems. My friend, the Harvard professor Edward O. Wilson, has assured me that few people are prepared to study the bigger picture in science.

So this is where I am today. I live in Canada now, in a house my husband and I built in the midst of a large research garden of native plants and trees surrounded by 65 hectares (160 acres) of forest south of Ottawa, Ontario. I study what is all around me and I write, bringing together botany and biochemistry, aboriginal healing, traditional wisdom and Western medicine in my own particular vision in science. Most of my work is peer reviewed by university scientists and published by a university press for the world to use as foundational thinking, whether in medicine, biochemistry, physics or engineering. As luck would have it, my husband, Christian, educated in linguistics and mathematics, retired early, making us a team of two. His father, the late Hermann Wilhelm Kroeger, a deputy director at the Marshall Space Flight Center for NASA, was also one of my firm supporters.

My book *The Global Forest* was for general readers. It was my attempt to reawaken people to the deep connection we have with trees. As E.O. Wilson

says, "To speak of trees you speak for all of nature."
I want to share my own life's mission to propagate
the mother trees of the world's forests and to save the
planet by replanting and tending such trees. In that
book I wanted to show people why human health,
the environment and trees are so inextricably linked.
Everywhere I went when I was talking about that
book, people asked me for ways in which they could
help with saving and planting trees, but also for any
little tips and practical wisdom I could offer to help
them recalibrate their lives so they could live more
harmoniously with nature. That is when I decided
to write *The Sweetness of a Simple Life.*

This book is full of wisdoms to restore your life
and help you connect to the natural world. Most
probably, you rarely take time to think about this
larger environment, but it is directly connected to
your health and welfare. Nature provides the food
you eat, so slow down and take a bite. Savour it for
its singular simplicity. If you get that far in this
collection, I will tell you more about my bigger
mission: saving the global forests for your children
and your children's children. We can do it together
by simplifying our lives and making our homes

healthier. I ask only one thing of you: give me your hand. Hold on tightly. I will not let go. We are on a mission to help nature, our world and our only home. Together, we will succeed.

CAUTION

I speak about medicines, sickness and hope in this book. Any advice I give is the same I use for myself to make my life run smoothly. But remember, the decisions I make on a daily basis are backed by thirteen years of university training and a lifetime of experience.

If you have a health problem, consult your medical practitioners for a solution. Then go home and apply common sense.

Part I

HEALTH AND FOOD

Turn on the tap in your kitchen and let the water flow for a minute. Then smell it. The water should smell clean. Taste it. The water should be neutral on the tongue. Look at it. The water should be clear, without traces of sediment.

In some places in the world, ancient water from the deep underground aquifers brings us hydrogen sulphide and calcium from the underlying dolomitic rock. Hydrogen sulphide carries a vague smell of rotten eggs, and calcium's presence is seen as precipitate in kettles and toilets. The vapours of hydrogen sulphide will off-gas on their own. Calcium in water is good for bone and teeth formation, and for the heart, in humans and animals alike. These waters were and still are used for spa treatments.

Next, go into the bathroom and look at yourself in the mirror. Smile. Keep that smile for everybody you meet during the day. It is the first offering of the heart to family and strangers alike. The afterglow of a smile will remain with the people you have met. It is a good thing to do, and likely the cheapest way to improve your well-being.

Now carry on to my essays on health and food. You will find a treasury of little wisdoms. Pick out those that speak to you and adopt them as a habit. Each act, in time, will become your character, forming your destiny—that of living an uncluttered, healthier life with more time for yourself and everyone else.

Twenty-Minute Pancreas

Walking is wonderful for your pancreas...

When I was a university student in the United States, I hitched my Irish accent under my arm with my books on advanced math and chemistry and headed for the labs. Every single morning a simmering sun rose early with me and the shadows of the night stepped back from the day to join the pine trees. A smell of tar held hands with the road and would not mix with the peach blossoms of the fields. A frisson of pine needles swept the air clean ahead of me and motioned me on my way.

Cars stopped to offer me a lift. The drivers worried about me walking alone. Some told me it was not proper: nobody walked around the campus. It was not done. These drivers, all of whom I knew, could not understand that I enjoyed my walk. Some laid both hands on the rim of the steering wheel in resignation, considering me to be too backward to understand the meaning of human transport. Others just shook their heads. Many more remained polite, but told me that what I was doing was definitely dangerous. They feared for my safety.

But I loved the sun, the heat, the rain and even the cold. This was my only exercise of the day. I needed it.

I joked that if everybody in the United States were to stop walking, they and their children would become fat. Babies might even be born with short, vestigial legs. Some would become so large that they could not bend down to see their toes. If they stopped walking their brains would grow sluggish and they would not be able to think for themselves. Diabetes would set in. Maybe even the younger children would get it. (At the time, I was only joking, though I was later proved to be on the mark.)

As I walked to and from the labs I began to imagine a world without exercise. Skin tone would go and people would become pallid. Children would lose their interest in being young. Men would go bald earlier. Women's hair would lose its natural shine of health and go limp. IQ would drop.

Exercise is part of living. It is one of the great pleasures of being alive. It is free. It is simple.

Walking conditions both body and mind. It quickens the circulation, forcing the heart to pump more blood. A pumping heart is a healthy heart. More blood flow means more oxygen delivery to the nooks and crannies of the body. The pancreas is just one of those nooks hanging from the large intestine, ready to fire off bullets of insulin as needed. All the pancreas requires to stay healthy is a little exercise. Twenty minutes a day is all that's necessary. You could call it a twenty-minute walk or simply a twenty-minute pancreas. Take your pick.

Get Some Sleep

Good sleep at night gives health to your day . . .

Shakespeare was no biochemist, but he hit the subject on the head when in *Macbeth* he wrote about "Sleep that knits up the ravell'd sleeve of care."

The act of sleep, like the act of eating, is no longer treasured. Sleep has lost its value in a busy world. Every single human being needs the safety of the night in slumber, in dreaming and in rest. Those who do not get this sleep will surely die young.

I had a friend called Adam. He was from Poland. He had been imprisoned in Siberia where, night after night as he fell asleep, he was woken up by brilliant lights shining into his face. His sleep cycle was broken. After his release he never regained a normal sleep pattern, although as an engineer, he was still brilliant. Sleep deprivation is a form of torture, first of the mind and then of the body. It throws a long shadow on health. This form of torture breaks people down, ultimately destroying their health. It killed Adam, though it took thirty years.

I was with him during his dying days. The only comfort he felt in these sleepless hours was my speaking to him the Latin prayers of his religion. The soft cadence of the words and the echo of their memory seemed to give him a form of rest. It activated in him a special form of prophecy. He would go into a reverie and tell me the future. He certainly understood the past. He died with happiness in his poor sleepless breast and a smile in his aged, waterlogged eyes.

There is in every brain a chemical curtain that divides up the night from the day. When this curtain closes, it shuts down the physical activity of the body, releasing it into a form of deep relaxation called sleep, while opening up the neural pathways into that strange form of freedom, the dream. The curtain is made up of a human hormone called melatonin. It is produced deep in the brain in a region of the pineal gland and possibly in another site. Melatonin travels to and binds itself for action in the part of the brain called the hypothalamus. From this kingpin position, melatonin affects the day and night cycle of the body. Because melatonin is so important, it is finely regulated by a number of proteins, one of which is a tiny piece of peptide composed of amino acids.

Melatonin is the timekeeper of the human body, and is sensitive to light. The clock is the sun and the seasons. When the body is exposed to light, very little melatonin is manufactured. But as the light changes to full darkness the chemical curtain of melatonin increases to produce the profound drowsiness prior to sleep. All during the hours of darkness, melatonin protects both body and mind. It protects the body against cancers, too. A lack of sleep appears to increase the risk factor of cancer in some people. Melatonin also seems to help regulate blood sugar. A lack of decent sleep and exposure to light during sleep opens the melatonin chemical curtain to type 2 diabetes. In addition, a body without adequate sleep expresses itself in a weakened immune system, in depression and in obesity.

There are household remedies that can help the natural flow of melatonin in the body. Eat fruit, especially bananas, during the day for the essential amino acids to make melatonin. Before sleep eat a tiny piece of hard cheese, which will take a while to dissolve in stomach acids, or take one teaspoon of high-fat natural yogurt. Both will coat the lining of the stomach and make calcium available to the pancreas. Then turn off all the screens and the lights, every single one, at least one to two hours before bed. Meditate or fill your mind with good, heartwarming thoughts. Relax the tensions of your body. Wake up in eight hours' time to a bright new day of well-being. Feel the flush of health run through your body. Now, that's real.

Red Wine

Red wine is a potent medicine . . .

My love affair with *Vitis*, the grape, has been ongoing for most of my life. I became a black sheep a long time ago. A friend of my family, Lady Jane Grey, took me in hand before one of her celebrations in the royal borough of Kensington in London, England. She insisted that I, like all children, should be given a drop of wine. It was healthy and she firmly believed that it would stop a child from becoming an alcoholic as an adult. She presented me with a small, hand-blown, green goblet from her collection, so I could better appreciate the merits of the wine itself. I kept it for years until it broke.

Later, when I was a student, my mutton instincts led me to the Napa Valley in California. Somehow, by accident, I found the location of one of the top vineyards there, the growing area a 1.6 hectare (4 acre) affair. The owner and vintner carefully stored and aged his Cabernet Sauvignon progeny year after year. I found myself in his back room with a wine glass in my hand. He carefully poured out his gold. While we were deliberating on its delights, a mink-clad lady entered his shop. She bought a case. The price took my breath away. I watched her leave with a list to the portside because of the weight of the emeralds she was wearing.

I carefully store away in my mind every morsel of knowledge I acquire about *Vitis*. Grapes of different *Vitis* cultivars were a wedding gift from my scientific friends and colleagues who worked with me in medicine. They joined Christian and me in picking and trouncing, in making our first vintage of red wine from the Fredonia black grape from a small vineyard planted at the head of the vegetable garden.

The wild grape in my garden, *Vitis riparia*, also known as the frost grape, gets my affection also. This Canadian wild plant is magnificent beyond belief. From one pip it will produce brown bullwood that will support a yearly mass of green tendrils that can climb to the top of any mature tree. This swag of growth produces a matrix of blooms composed of tiny green to white blossoms that are exquisitely fragrant in the late spring. The scent is heavy like magnolia and seems to settle around the vine in a vapour. This smell attracts wildlife in prodigious numbers to feed and fertilize the flowers. Grapes are formed during the summer months and turn from green to black in October.

Songbirds use the wild grape, grooming its green acreage for food. They settle there, nest and stay. Other larger birds use this vine to escape from the even larger predatory birds. When frost touches the wild grape harvest, the fruit sugars re-form and fermentation happens in situ. The larger game birds move in to drink and get drunk. They form the circus of the fall with their tricks and antics.

The grape is a remarkable plant. It supports itself by growing two sets of adventitious roots. The upper set scrounges the soil for food latterly. The lower roots plunge as deeply as they can and will interface with the rocks for the minerals that the plant needs. The grapes produced later on in the season will reflect these minerals as a sweeter taste on the tongue.

The aboriginal peoples of North America have eaten the fruit of the wild grape for 40,000 years in a most interesting way, and they taught the pioneers to do the same thing. After the first damaging frost in September to November, they will pick a good-looking bunch of grapes. They will cradle the bunch in their cupped hand and, one by one, pick each grape off the bunch and eat it. They suck the skins before they swallow the grape, then spit out the seeds. A child will play with the grape longer, often latching his or her tongue through the skin. The medicine that is in the grape is extracted in this way and goes directly into the body on a wave of digestive juices. Aboriginal healers use the grape to cure hiccoughs, for renal cleansing and for hair restoration following fever. As a hair restorative, vine sap is boiled with the yellow-flowered barren strawberry, *Waldsteinia fragarioides*, and used as a rinse and a scalp massage to strengthen the growth of the hair on the head.

It was noticed that French and Italian men who drank wine daily enjoyed cardiac health into old age, this despite liberal doses of foie gras and escargots drowned in a vat of butter. In 1995, the biochemistry of the cultivated grape was examined for the health value of wine. One biochemical popped out of the mixture: resveratrol. Technically resveratrol is a phytoalexin or a stress hormone produced by the grapevine in response to injury or poor growing conditions. Grapes, because of their annual leaf growth, are prone to fungal infection. The vine produces resveratrol to combat these pathogens in the skin of the grape and around the seeds inside the grape to protect the future of the species.

It seems that resveratrol has a direct action on the heart by enabling blood to freely flow through the circulatory system. The biochemical has a natural action on the blood cells themselves, keeping each one separate. This separation is vital to prevent clotting, which, in turn, is beneficial to all those suffering from coronary heart disease. It also appears that resveratrol has an ability to interfere with the life of a cancer cell by inhibiting its growth, making resveratrol a powerful anti-cancer agent, one that is now securely under examination as a drug of the future.

Strangely enough, resveratrol has been around as a medicine for millennia and modern science had never noticed. It is the active ingredient of many species of knotweed, *Polygonum*, which is a member of the buckwheat family. The Cree and Slave nations of northern Canada have used water knotweed, *Polygonum amphibium*, for its medicine for generations.

It has been used across the Arctic and down into the Kamchatka peninsula of Russia by the aboriginal peoples there as the giant knotweed, *P. sachalinense*—a forage plant. In Asia it is the powdered medicine known as *kojo-kon*, which has been used to treat the blood, heart and liver.

Another medicinal bonus from resveratrol comes from its plant regulator effect. It has an anti-aging function in the human cell. Only time will tell how good it is.

In any case, Lady Jane was onto something big. And I listened when I was young. I toast her memory with one small glass of red wine a day. One such glass will keep you fit and young. Less is always more when it comes to wine and health.

PHYTO FIX

More medicine, and hope, from plants . . .

I was shown a different slice of life as a child. I was taught the cures held in the hand of nature. If I had a wart, my great-uncle would produce a potato and slice it in half, cut out a hollow, and place a pinch of rock salt into it. Then he set the potato in the light and waited twenty-four hours. He would say to me, "Let me cure your wart." He dabbed the solution that had formed in the hollow of the potato on my finger and the wart disappeared. It was an old Irish cure, and many more cures from the ancient medicine of the Druids were handed down to me.

I went on to study medical biochemistry in the sixties when vitamins had become the stars. We were told that vitamin C could cure the common cold. Proteins were on the stage, too, with their eight essential amino acids, such as tryptophan, the precursor to serotonin. Tryptophan is now used in the treatment of depression, schizophrenia and other neuropsychiatric disorders of the mind. The ability of carbohydrates to form polymeric strings of structure caused much excitement for the organic chemists. All three fatty acids, known to be essential for human health, were still out of sight, waiting in the wings. They are extremely difficult to study, but they are now moving toward the spotlight because of the epidemic of obesity in our children who are not getting the right kinds of fat in their diets.

Recently a stranger has stepped into centre stage. The newcomer is a class of biochemicals from the plant world called phytochemicals. These players are complex and exciting because they open up so many possibilities for new medicines and different approaches to treatments of diseases.

Phyta is Greek for plant. A phytochemical is a biochemical that comes from a plant source. The plant may be algae, fungus, moss, lichen, a fern, a flower, or an evergreen or deciduous tree. The potential of the phytochemical world is enormous.

The DNA of a tree, any tree, is more complex than that of a human being. This DNA is the baseline regulator of the thing we call life and it has to be governed by a very tight set of rules. Phytochemicals set the ground rules for a vegetable, a flower or a tree's behaviour. A Boston lettuce will not grow to 30 metres (100 feet) and a mushroom will not turn green like a leaf because of the limits set by the phytochemicals. In a plant like a lettuce or a carrot, phytochemicals are produced in greatest abundance when the maturing vegetable is ready to be harvested.

Truth for a phytochemical is stranger than fiction. The phytochemicals that act like plant hormones, regulating the life of the plant through the various stages from birth to death, seem to have a similar ability to fine-tune the human body. When eaten in food, some phytochemicals can act as serious metabolic regulators. Some screen the human cell for diseases such as cancer and eliminate the cancerous cells in a variety of ways, one of which is to shut down the network of blood vessels that feed and water the growing tumour. These phytochemicals are the ellagic acid compounds in small fruits and nuts. Others, such as anthocyanidins, which provide the colouring of fruits and vegetables, shut down DNA synthesis. Proanthocyanidins in small fruits and berries reduce the manufacture of the human hormone estrogen, for both men and women, thus slowing the rate at which cancer cells grow.

Limonene is another fascinating anti-cancer phytochemical. Many plants and trees manufacture this phytochemical when they are flowering and looking for pollinators. The flower releases a chemical carte de visite in its scent or perfume. The scent must lift to travel the airways. Limonene supplies that lift like the wings of a bird. The molecular structure of limonene is like a tiny windmill and functions like one, too.

Many mushroom phytochemicals are lentinans. They are powerfully active as anti-tumour agents and also stimulate the immune system to fight for the body's greater health. The aboriginal peoples of North America certainly knew about mushrooms because they made a point of collecting the continent's best of the mushroom world, the morel, *Morchella esculenta*, from the riches of the forest floor every summer.

Phytochemicals are found in herbs such as basil, coriander, cumin, lovage, parsley and rosemary. They are found in the colouring of all vegetables, especially in the bright heritage tomatoes returning to the food markets. Potatoes all carry different colours in the cortex of their skins, especially the heritage species. Apples, too. The list goes on for the kitchen and the cook. The message for the daily menu is diversity, because if you eat a broad range of brightly coloured foods, you are assured of a higher volume of phytochemicals in the food that you consume to protect your daily health.

In some ways, I have come full circle from the child I was. A few years ago I addressed the Assembly of First Nations. I was invited to speak about the importance of the forests of North America. A medicine man said to me, "The plants will unfold their medicines when the need for them will arise." I think of the vast number of phytochemicals waiting to be studied and I am happy for the hope they carry for us all. The biodiversity in the plant kingdom hoards a treasure trove of medicines for cures we are only just beginning to understand. But these cures could be gone tomorrow through the careless cutting of our forests.

Sea Food

The sea is an ancient source of good nutrition . . .

There are real health foods out there, vital to the maintenance of a healthy body and mind. One particular food is the oldest food source on the planet. It has always been picked from the wild, from the seashore. The food is seaweed. Edible seaweeds grow in intertidal zones in bays and estuaries where the tide meets the currents of the seas or freshwater rivers. The sea teems with life in these places due, in part, to the increased mineral content of the seawater itself, produced by erosion. The minerals in turn act as catalysts for the enzymes of plant life. These minerals can vary from gold to iron, and are needed by the human body.

In the last few centuries a form of sea farming was adapted to increase the yield of the crop. The fishermen of Japan, Korea and China initiated this practice by sticking oak branches into the sea floor and interweaving them to create strainers for the rich seawater. In the small eddies made by the branches, seaweeds were able to germinate from mobile spores that settled there, putting down rooting holdfasts into the wood as anchors. From these small beginnings large seaweeds were able to grow, absorbing rich nutrients into their growing thalli or bodies. The fishermen went out in their boats to hand cut and harvest the seaweed. Their crop always sold out.

Seaweeds are algae. Most algae live in the ocean, requiring salt water to survive. There are some on land and in fresh water, too. Algae come in all shapes and sizes, just like the plants that grow on land. There are tiny algae that live in silicon boxes, enamelled with art deco designs of nature. And there are algae that form kelp forests, growing and swaying with the movement of water and covered with sea life. Edible seaweeds are somewhere in between the big and small.

The health benefits from edible seaweeds are extraordinarily high. Seaweeds come in a rainbow of colours—greens, yellows, reds and browns—all of which are, in reality, beneficial biochemical polymeric sugars that can be used both inside the body as food or outside it in cosmetics. That rainbow of colours is also used by marine botanists to classify algae.

Seaweeds have a definite edge as a health food, matching the electrolyte balance in the blood. Human blood is always on the move, being the transportation system of the body. This active transport requires wheels, made not of rubber but of ions. These ions, also called electrolytes, give blood the electricity it needs for give-and-take at the capillary wall. People must eat ions, such as sodium, aluminum, iron, iodine, gold, magnesium and manganese, in trace amounts, to maintain a healthy body.

In the past, island nations had health rituals using seaweeds. The ancient Celts took their health food from the sea with great respect, and Druidic physicians directed the use of algae carefully. A favourite was a little, red, curly seaweed found fastened on the rocks at the farthest reach of the low tide. This ancient medicine, the famous carrageen moss, *Chondrus crispus*, was collected in baskets and boiled into a jelly for its complex mixtures of sugars. It was the original antibiotic used by the Irish to treat tuberculosis. It stands now as one of the historical desserts of old Irish cuisine, eaten these days as a health food.

Nowadays, sea farming has grown and science has entered the picture. In Asia, kelp farmers sink bamboo poles into the mud. Net curtains are draped from the poles and the net is seeded with shells. These white shells become the havens for a part of the life cycle of algae called the sporophyte generation. This mass of plants is fertilized in situ by nitrogen fertilizers that slowly flush out of hanging pots interspersed in the net curtain.

The plants are harvested by boat and air-dried on land where they form great sheets of vegetable matter that is cut and then folded, packaged and labelled for market.

One species of edible seaweed well known on the east coast of North America is laver. This same seaweed is called *Porphyra*, its Latin name, on the western shores of Europe. In Japan, China and Korea, it is sold as nori, where it is harvested from late November into March when the seawater is higher in nitrogen. Nori is a plum-coloured algae with large, flat, mucilaginous leaves that are washed and then chopped and made into a liquid soup. It is poured over porous mats, then dried like a linen sheet. The food value of nori is extraordinary. A serving contains half again the vitamin C of an orange. It is 30 percent protein and full of complex sugars and mineral salts, especially iodine. Nori protects the thyroid, enabling this glandular organ to make selenoproteins, which are necessary for reproduction; when eaten with wheat germ, it protects against degenerative muscle diseases.

Another sea plant called kombu is a favourite in Japan. This brown algae grows in deep, rich seawater, and carries biochemicals that stimulate the sensitivity of the taste buds to sweet, sour, bitter and salty. Kombu also contains a high level of iodine, plus sugars and proteins that can clean the body of radioactive strontium. This seaweed is known as edible kelp in other parts of the world, and in Latin as *Laminaria saccharina japonica*. It is found in spots off the west coast of Canada and is extensively sea-farmed, especially on Hokkaido, the northern island of Japan. Kombu is dried, then powdered and drunk as a seaweed tea. It is used in soups, pickled, or shredded as an edible decoration. The most common place you would encounter it in Canada is in the wrap of sushi.

But probably the most important sea plant that is sea-farmed is wakame, a sea vegetable of Korea and

Japan. Its Latin name is *Undaria pinnatifida*. This brown kelp contains a pigment called fucoxanthin, which is related to vitamin A. This pigment can help oxidize or burn fat tissue that collects around the major organs. Wakame is an anti-obesity health food as, to a lesser extent, are all the seaweeds. They fire up the thyroid and burn fat, leaving you leaner and healthier in body and mind.

Cancer Prevention

Some vegetables protect us from cancer . . .

Chinese greens, or bok choi, are a member of the cabbage family that, for centuries, have lived a simple life in the gardens of China, Japan and Korea, and graced tables there. Bok choi, with its mild aftertaste of mustard, is a favourite vegetable of the Asian cook, and marries perfectly with the flavour of soya sauce. When young, it fills the hand and is sometimes called a baby bunch. The snow-white, broad petioles are added to many Korean dishes to blend a succulent freshness into the garlic-laced meat.

Bok choi is also known as pak choi. The plant is *Brassica rapa* or *B. chinensis*. This disease-resistant, healthy vegetable has many forms, all of which have been developed for a shorter day and early maturation. Bok choi seeds are small, round and black. A package costs a few dollars. It takes just a second to open and less again to broadcast them into the garden. Bok

choi seeds roll into the tiny cracks in the earth.
They settle in to wait for the frost of the spring or
fall. The seeds require cooler temperatures to trigger
the end of dormancy. Then they decide to grow.

The miracle anti-carcinogenic molecule in
bok choi is called dithiolethione. It is found in
the forest-green leaves. As the plant matures, the
amount of the molecule increases. Therefore,
the more mature bok choi better protects against
cancer. A taste of the raw greens unveils the
extraordinary medicine. On the tongue the leaves
produce a crisp tang from the sulphur in the
molecule. There are three atoms of sulphur that
form sulphur bridges in the cells of the body. The
architectural arrangement is very strong, and the
body finds them extremely useful.

Modern medicine is busy exploring and
understanding this molecule. There are more like
it out there in the chemistry of the cabbage family.
They are found in kimchi, which is fermented
Chinese cabbage, *B. pekinensis*. They are also in
sauerkraut, the fermented glory of Germany. Both
are now known as probiotic foods or foods that help
the beneficial bacteria of the human gut because they

are fermented, which adds to the ecology of the human digestive system.

Twenty-five years ago I invested in a packet of bok choi seeds. I rolled them into the garden soil. Ever since, the return has been great. I watch for the cruciform, four green leaves, of the tiny tots. They come immediately to the call of spring. I leave two plants to grow into three-foot-tall mother plants. We eat the rest. The honeybees always find the bright yellow flowers on the top. The bees and butterflies drink the nectar and fertilize the flowers. In a week or two, small, round and black bok choi seeds roll themselves out of the maturing seed capsules into the garden in front of my eyes . . . and I wait in wonder for the cool days of another spring.

Chocolate Chips

Chocolate and blood have a lot in common . . .

I will admit to a passion for chocolate, but my passion is in the garden. I simply love the smell of chocolate as it wafts about our North American Medicine Walk, with all of the memory of taste and the tingle of excitement the fragrance engenders. The Medicine Walk is the part of my garden where I collect many native medicinal plants and a few favourite imports. The smells come from the edible chocolate vine, *Akebia trifoliata*, which swings its black flowers from on high, dangling over the northern *allée*. And also from the black peonies, *Paeonia lactiflora* 'Chocolate Soldier,' and all of the dark-flowered siblings I have bred, breathing out fumes of chocolate.

To me, chocolate and blood have a lot in common. Both substances can move and flow. Chocolate comes from the cacao bean, which is the large seed of the

cacao tree, *Theobroma cacao*. This small evergreen
is an understory tree of Central and South America.
It loves the wet lowlands of the tropical rainforests.
The yellow flowers growing from the trunk bear a
30-centimetre (12-inch) fruit filled with a sweet,
mucilaginous pulp in which the cacao seeds are
embedded. The fruit is called a pod. It is pollinated
by midges and looks like a long squash. The tree
represented the financial system of the Aztecs who
used the bean as currency. A slave could be bought
with one hundred beans!

Cacao beans are high in fats. These fats are part of the
seed's treasury. They are the endosperm riches, which
is like the colostrum in breast milk, enabling a young
tree to grow in wet ground. The mother tree feeds this
protective battery of chemicals into each seed. These
chemicals are flavonoid phenolics that shield the fats
and prevent them from becoming rancid.

As luck would have it, in 1828 the seeds of
Theobroma cacao were passed to a Dutch manufacturer
named Coenraad Johannes van Houten. This
gentleman quickly invented a method to express
much of the fat from the cacao seed, then added sugar,
making it more palatable and digestible for the

European market. The "food of the gods" received the adoration it deserved and chocolate was born, dark and rich and flavourful.

When you eat a piece of dark chocolate, the same flavonoid phenols that the mother tree placed in her seeds criss-cross your tongue, melting in flavour, and travel happily into the stomach, where they pass through the stomach wall, taking just two hours to hit the bloodstream as it surges along. Human blood behaves like an oil because it is composed of special oil-bearing proteins called lipoproteins. One of these attracts the immediate attention of the flavonoid phenols of the chocolate, a low-density lipoprotein or LDH.

The LDH is known as "bad" cholesterol because it is a floater. This lipoprotein attaches itself to the intima or inner wall of large arteries and settles there, causing arterial plaque. As the deposits of lipoprotein increase, the diameter of the artery decreases, so much so that it produces cardiovascular diseases, one of which is arteriosclerosis. With a reduced flow-way in the artery, the heart must pump harder to push the same volume of required blood through these narrow arteries, causing high blood pressure. High blood pressure can, over time, lead to all kinds of difficulties in the body.

The other lipoprotein in the blood is a high-density form, HDL. This lipoprotein is the good fraction of cholesterol. The emulsifying action of HDL facilitates the flow of the blood and its ability to carry all the round, doughnut-shaped red blood cells and their helpers, keeping them on target. This easy flow oxygenates the cells of the body and carries away the detritus to collection depots for excretion.

Dark, rich chocolate comes to the rescue of blood. The flavonoid phenolics that are present to preserve the fat in the beans do the same thing for the low-density lipoproteins of the blood. The flavonoid phenolics protect these lipoproteins from going "bad" because they are strong antioxidants. This is why chocolate is good for the heart and the circulation in general. Not a lot of chocolate, just a little piece is good once in a while during the course of the week.

Meanwhile, I stick to my Medicine Walk to smell the chocolate, which also happens to be a bronchodilator, opening the body's airways. It adds to my pleasure as a gardener, especially when I walk outside to visit my black, chocolate-scented peonies when they are in full bloom. I always bend my head to smell their wonderful fragrance, and to get my chocolate top-up for the day. Inevitably, I am left with a well-pollinated bright yellow nose as a rich reward.

Bee's Knees

Beef broth will keep your aches and pains away . . .

The baby boomers are bulging through the population, like a supercharged fetus in a skin 'n' bone female. The boomers had flower power. Then they had professions and political power, and now they have aches and pains, lots of them. Pity them. Please. This is new to them. This time they all have the equality they wished for, because pain knows no gender.

Boomers had the thrill of the Pill and, in a way, they are paying for it now. They have had the benefit of very little generational wisdom, advice passed from Mom to daughters and Dad to sons. So the generation gap is great. Birth control delayed pregnancy and child rearing for many until a point when the grandparents were too old for knowledge transfer. Wisdom is lost. And the youth are, too.

For boomers, menopause has come like a thief in the night and stolen their restless days. Hair has gone

and wrinkles walk in. Hormonal supplements are
plied to aid sagging skin and everything else that
needs a tad of starch. Drinking water is full of
medicinal estrogens and xenochemicals that mimic
human reproductive hormones. They have another
go at the gonads and wash out the womb. This
hormonal water is payback time for the boomers.
They get a double dose of pain. Hormone molecules
affect the joints of the fingers, the hands, the feet, the
toes and the tendons. The knees give out and the hips
follow suit. The back is stiff and the weight of the
head wears out the neck. The linkages that connect
all the bones of the skeleton are a form of biological
rubber. This rubber is kept supple and working by
the reproductive hormones of the body.

Women are well aware of biological rubber, the way
it opens the birthing canal and expanding connective
tissue so that the fetus can slip its way through. But
older feet never come back to their chic shape and rib
cages are forever wider. And waists are, too.

Biological rubber is what makes the skeleton
work. The rubber is a mucopolysaccharide made
up of connecting units of chondroitin 4-sulphate
and chondroitin 6-sulphate, the most abundant

polymeric sugars of the body. They occur with and are attached to the skeleton and in all of the soft, moving and connective tissue of the body. These sugar polymers connect with protein in cartilage to form a matrix with bounce and movement almost identical to the reinforced rubber found in the tires of your car or tractor.

This biological rubber can be replaced. As the body ages the rubber is sometimes worn a little, frayed at the edges, especially if the skeleton is carrying too much weight on the bones. Weight causes extra wear and the first sign of wear is on the connecting rubber between the bones. A cheap and healthy way to supplement these rubber cushions between your bones is something your grandmother should have told you: a good bowl of hot homemade soup made from beef broth. It has all the ingredients to stop your aches and pains in your knees, fingers, feet, hips, neck and back.

So go to your butcher and buy some beef bones. Make sure the bones are organic, from local beef. Ask questions and if you do not get the right answer, go to another store. Usually, I order ahead. My order is for ten pounds of bones that are wrapped in three to four lots. I freeze these. The bones should be big, thick marrowbones with some meat on them. Go home and wash the bones to remove bone chips. Put them in a large pot with cold water to cover them by at least one inch. Bring to the boil. Then slowly simmer the bones for forty-eight hours, adding more cold water to keep the bones covered. Cool the beef stock.

The cooled beef stock should set like a jelly. The better the bones, the greater the gel set. This gel contains the chondroitin sulphate that has been extracted from the bones. It should have a light brown colour. It is one of the best forms of nutrition for people with osteoarthritis because it has calcium as well as chondroitin sulphate in its solution. In the past, in many countries, this broth was used as a food for invalids both young and old who were recovering from sickness.

I freeze the entire pot of stock, then remove the hard surface of snow-white fat. I save this pure fat, or suet, bagging it for the freezer again, and use it to make bird cakes for winter feeders. If you keep hens, they simply love pecking at suet over the winter months.

Then I warm the stock a little, only enough so I can remove the bones and peel off any meat, which goes back into the pot. Then I freeze the stock in batches. One litre (1 quart) of beef stock makes 6 litres (6 quarts) of wonderful soup with added vegetables.

I keep the bones from the stockpot, wash them off, and save them in a large jute bag that I store in my garden shed. These bones become my bone meal for use in planting holes for my trees and shrubs. Nut trees, fruit trees and grapevines require a constant source of available calcium to successfully produce a nut, fruit or grape crop year after year. Large beef bones act as a calcium, phosphorous and potash source, which feeds the soil for twenty-five years.

The biological rubber, or chondroitin sulphate, is the real cushion of the body, and it is the sulphur from the sulphate that is the action-packed element of it all: the bounce. I remember old people in Ireland being described with just the right amount of give and balance in their footsteps as having "the bee's knees."

Marriage Menopause

The hormones of attraction change at menopause . . .

Apart from time, marriage is often the most
precious thing to most human beings. Marriage
creates the tribe: the moms, the dads, the aunts, the
uncles, the sisters and brothers and, of course, the
grandparents. But few understand the long game
of marriage.

The villain of the story is DNA. All of us have those
little sprigs of knowledge in each of our cells. They
create the human condition. All DNA comes in twos,
like the heavenly twins. But for reproduction, in the
egg or in the sperm, the sprigs are found only as one.
This is known in science as the haploid state. The
cells have unwound the DNA and wait to make two
again in the parental bed. Mortals travelling through
life in steerage have faced down poverty or worse for
the one partner who will make him or her happy.

The egg of a woman with one sprig of DNA meets

the sperm of a man with his sprig of DNA . . . and all of the world becomes one in that moment of meeting and mating. The two sprigs of DNA are each half of a helix. At mating, a new double helix is formed, accompanied by the pleasures of endorphins. Kings have lost their kingdoms and queens have lost their heads for these sexual pleasures.

But marriage is more . . . much more. Marriage has a menopause, a time when the old grandmother shakes her head and says, "The gilt has gone," or if you happen to be Irish, "The icing has disappeared from the wedding cake." By this she means that one or the other partner has lost interest in the marriage bed. Or perhaps both have.

The same little sprig of DNA of the egg or the sperm that caused you such consternation when you were a teen and such erotic pleasure when you were first married is now up to other biochemical tricks. These tricks usually strike when you are in your forties or fifties. Some unfortunates meet the menopause wall in their thirties. For some males, the limit has been reset to the sixties and beyond, with a little dose of invigorating drugs from the bastion of modern medicine.

At menopause for a man and for a woman, the body experiences a change of hormonal tide. This tide had come rushing in to bathe each cell with youth until a balance was achieved. Now this balance changes and all of the biochemistry associated with it does, too, creating the new horizon of life.

Women lose their reproductive capacity. With this change comes weird wonders for some: a pain in a big toe, a pain in the tibia or larger bone of the leg while drinking a glass of red wine, night sweats, day sweats, sleeplessness and memory loss, anger, angst and anxiety.

Men go bald. Their wives become transparent, and younger women lithesome and apparent. Some men turn into couch potatoes while others jump generations and choose a child bride, even start another family. The grandad-daddy cares for children he will never know as adults.

A lack of understanding of marriage menopause can cause separation and divorce. In many cases, divorce causes estrangements and hatred among the children, too. The family suffers and can never be put right again.

A year ago my husband, Christian, and I were in

Ireland for a number of media events, one of which was to speak in a tiny, ninth-century stone church built by the last high king of Ireland. It was in County Clare, in a remote part of Ireland. The organizers, my husband and I shared a large house on the shores of Lough Derg.

During breakfast, I struck up a conversation with an organizer. One thing led to another, as happens when you are looking out at sacred waters with a gentle mist rising up from them. Lough Derg seemed to relax everybody and encouraged us to linger over our tea and chat.

She was in an abject state of misery. She did not know what to do about her marriage. Everything was going wrong. Life itself was sweeping her away in opposite directions from her teenage daughters and her husband. She did not know which way to turn. And she turned to me for advice. It was safe. I was a stranger. I could offer something neutral.

This woman seemed typical of the new Ireland. She was a professional and so was her husband. Money was not a source of worry. They had a city house and a country one, too. The Lough Derg property in which we were staying was hers. In her state of confusion she decided to remain in the country house while her husband and her school-going girls lived in Dublin.

She was not sleeping well. She woke up many times a night in a state of anxiety. She felt her mind was going because she could not recall the names of people she'd known all her life. There were many other things during her daily routine that she could not recall either. Simple things like sugar and butter. She would go into one room to get something and forget what it was she wanted while she was there. She would stand and think, looking around. Nothing came. "Sex," she laughed at me. "I have no interest. My husband has no attraction for me anymore." She was seeing another man.

I suggested to her that she was menopausal. The hormonal balance that guided her life in her twenties was in flux. She was now forty-five. Her estrogen levels were changing; hence the lack of interest in sex with her husband and the memory loss that went with everyday living. She brightened up visibly.

Then I pointed out that an estrogen drop, in my opinion, is a protective shield for a woman. It comes at a time in the life cycle when the rates of problem births and mental retardation in babies are on the increase. An estrogen drop is a biochemical message to the reproductive system to take a permanent holiday. Time off, in other words. It is not the end of the world, just the beginning of another.

It is a time when love between a man and woman has time to ferment into another form of security: that of being cherished. Memory does come back, because the body has its own form of balance or harmony and neural pathways do pick up the slack. And the best news of all, two people age better than one. Better for the children, too.

The beautiful Celt went back to her husband and her teenage girls. She returned to mend the marriage. Our hormones change at menopause. We are all caught in that tide at some point in our lives, sooner or later.

No Smoking

How to stop forever . . .

It is true that I married a cigarette. My husband smoked three packs a day, followed by the combustion of a pipe and his cigars. His personal production toward climate change was brought to a screeching halt when the lung squad visited his government office to do a lung capacity test on all those laying down their lives for the greater good of civil society.

Following this test, Christian must have had some pep left in his system because he popped like a rubber band up several flights of stairs to a colleague's office. On the landing he was stopped short by a severe fall of soot, which caused a fit of coughing and difficulty breathing. His lungs also produced some strange debris. I suspect that the small coloured bands of Cuban cigars were in the mix.

I rolled up my sleeves and went to work as quickly as possible, offering him a clean leaf on which I wrote a diet to help him stop smoking based on my biochemical knowledge.

Let me back the horse into the cart for a moment. Smoking is an extremely serious and powerful addiction. What makes the habit so difficult to break is that it interferes with a number of biochemical pathways in each cell of the body, even blood cells or erythrocytes. Tobacco contains nicotinic acid or nicotine, a biologically active component of a co-enzyme called nicotinamide adenine dinucleotide or NAD. This NAD is like a ball bearing to a working cell. It is the workhorse that moves hydrogen around, and is a vital hydrogen donor in the respiratory chain for total oxygen use.

As if this were not enough, the very act of smoking and breathing in the nicotine presses the hot button in the brain that releases endorphins—the pleasure centre of all that feels good and wonderful—so you don't wish to stop, even when you know smoking is not good for your long-term health.

Smoking ages the cells of the body, starving them of oxygen. The first ones to go are the cells in the gums, leading to periodontal disease. Teeth get loose and fall out. The heart and the circulation seem to be affected because the heart is the running organ of the body and if it stops for a break, you die or at best have a mild heart attack. The heart needs NAD with its full supply of oxygen. You cannot expect your cardiologist to be too pleased if you prop yourself up on your hospital pillow and ask for a smoke after a quadruple bypass. But this happens.

When Christian decided to quit I put him on a cleansing diet. Lots of water. I mean clean well water, fossil wild water if you like, fresh from the underground aquifer. Then I cut all stimulants like tea, coffee, alcohol and sugars out of his diet. Every day he swallowed an anti-stress pill, available over the counter, containing all of the B vitamins together with folic acid and a good dose of vitamin C. The B vitamin complex acts as a synergistic substitute to block the action of the tobacco's nicotine and to help with the anxiety of withdrawal. The vitamin C maintains the integrity and function of the walls of the blood vessels during withdrawal.

The food he ate was organic—all of it. Food that is produced non-organically is often contaminated with antibiotics and a host of horticultural chemicals that interfere with the body's defense system against withdrawal. He cut back on red meats, which are high in tryptophan, an amino acid that is a precursor to serotonin. Limiting the intake of tryptophan takes the edge off headaches and eases the slippery slope of withdrawal.

Eating salads, specifically watercress and fresh spinach with dressings of cold-pressed, virgin olive oil and balsamic vinegars, cleanses the body, as do meals consisting of a mixture of vegetables together with white meats or deep sea fish like cod, halibut, haddock, Greenland turbot, scallops and wild shrimp. The electrolyte balance of these seafoods matches the exacting balance of the body's lymph system. An electrolyte balance in seafood comes from a variety of ions, which are atoms that hold a positive or negative charge. They act as conductors in biochemical reactions in the body, feeding electrons and changing the quantum state. These non-metallic ions are removed from the smoker's body. They must be replaced by what can be gleaned in food.

I also added fresh fruit to the menu, especially ripe bananas for their high potassium and some readily available serotonin. If you can find fresh pawpaws, eat them: they have cellular healing properties called acetogenins. Ripe, fresh mangos are good, too.

Now Christian is reformed. He simply cannot bear the smell of cigarette smoke. Success can be this simple . . .

KITCHEN AID

Garlic and onions are more than just essential flavours . . .

O pen the fridge door and pull out the crisper drawer. I hope you will find an onion rolling around, shedding some of its layers as it sits in cold comfort waiting to be cut up into a stew or finely sliced to top a sandwich. To the cook, the onion is indispensable, as it was in the past and as it will be in the future.

The earliest written documentation of garlic and onions being used as medicine comes from the Chaldeans, who lived in ancient Babylonia, part of modern-day Iraq, around 5,000 years ago. It could quite safely be said that the pyramids of Egypt were built on garlic because the slaves were meted out a daily ration of fresh garlic to go with their bread, not so much to feed them as to maintain their health. A sick slave costs money, as the pharaohs' accountants well knew. Rome ran on garlic too.

The Roman Empire insisted that its legions partake of the luxury of garlic, fresh, of course.

The longest oral memory of the onion being used as medicine comes from northern Canada, where the medicine men of the Cree Nation from the boreal forest system used wild chives, *Allium schoenoprasum*, and the aboriginal peoples of eastern North America picked, ate and treasured the wild garlic, *A. canadense*, which grows in the rich humus of the floor of virgin deciduous forests. This garlic was used as a blood cleanser and spring panacea for millennia.

Today, the onion family, *Alliaceae*, is still good medicine, breathing sulphur to shield us from cancer. All of *Alliaceae*'s many members carry a medical biochemical, allicin, that can act as a bloodhound in the body, sniffing out pre-cancer cells. Allicin then breaks down again into more active pieces to get the job done properly, killing those cells on the spot.

Some members of the onion family are better equipped than others to kill cancer. At the top of the list is garlic, *Allium sativum*, locally grown and summer harvested, eaten throughout the year. Next on the crying list are the winter storage onions,

A. cepa. They can be red-, brown- or white-skinned. Red is the best because these onions have additional anthocyanidin phytochemicals that protect our health. The outside of the onion should feel perfectly dry to the hand and somewhat crisp, a sign that the internal layers of the onion are in perfect order. Then come the leeks, *A. ampeloprasum*, Porrum group, with a sweetened, mild flavour much beloved by the Welsh.

Trotting at the heels of the adult onions, the shallots, *A. ascalonicum*, hold a special place of honour in France. And then there is the darling of China and Korea, Chinese chives, *A. tuberosum*, with its flat long leaves and liquid garlic flavour. There is one pot herb, the Egyptian or tree onion, *A. cepa*, of the Proliferum group, that the Canadian pioneers would simply not be without because of its availability throughout late fall and early spring when nothing else was growing in the garden. All people now know about chives, *A. schoenoprasum*, a true Canadian plant, and bunching onions or scallions, *A. fistulosum*. They can be found in two colours; choose the red for its anthocyanidin content.

The crying factor in onion and in garlic is a simple biochemical called alliin, whose molecule holds an atom of sulphur. Alliin is extremely water-soluble and is released very quickly into the air when the garlic or onion is chopped. The cook gets the worst deal in the kitchen because he or she has to lean over the onion with a knife and gets the first wave of alliin into the eyes, the nose and mouth. This alliin may cause tears, but next time you are crying think of how that molecule is soon broken down to allicin and cancer protection is on its way.

There is a folklore tradition in Europe around the storage of garlic and onions. The garlic stems are usually braided and hung from a hook in the kitchen while it is slowly being used. The onions are stored in net bags and also hung. The heat from cooking continues to cure the outer skins while they hang. As the outer layers of both onion and garlic dry, they release alliin into the air. The amount is small, but ever present. This airborne alliin begins the inhibition of growth of cancer cells in all members of the household, adults, children, even pets. Then, when eaten, the garlic and onions become an active medicine in the body.

As well as inhibiting cellular cancer, the onion family reduces cholesterol and glucose in the bloodstream. Garlic in particular lowers elevated blood pressure and inhibits the aggregation of red blood cells that cause stroke. But there is one cautionary note: garlic works so well as a blood thinner that you shouldn't eat it in the twenty-four hours preceding any kind of surgery.

Alliin research continues to be in the headlines linked to treatment of hormone-stimulated cancers like breast and prostate cancer. Also, the alliin from onions, garlic and chives seems to stimulate the immune system and help people shed flus, colds and bronchitis more easily. The kitchen miracle at work.

Real Brain Food

The true omega . . .

I have a rare cherry tree planted outside of the kitchen door. It has spread its branches to cross the kitchen window. The tree is a heritage English morello cherry brought into North America by a pioneering family two hundred years ago. I even know where the original cherry seed came from—a little village in County Wexford, Ireland. Every summer cherry pies from this tree grace my table.

This spring I saw a magical event. The cherry was in full bloom. The cast of the sky was grey and it had been raining for a few days. The flowers were a startling white and looked like a cluster of stars. The green leaves had not yet unfurled, so the snowstorm of blossom was mine to admire.

Then a Baltimore oriole dropped into the picture, its brilliant orange a flame against the grey and white. The bird tipped its beak into the cup of one of the

flowers and drank the nectar-rich water greedily.
The bird emptied the flower and hopped to the next
one, staying until his hunger and thirst had gone.
The oriole had the deft ability of the acrobat, the
magic of movement.

Such coordination and beauty in this bird caught
me in a pearl of thought, about the length of time it
took to complete this act of evolution to the point of
perfection in the bird. Millions and millions of years.

An internal building block makes such movement
possible. I mean all movement: the thought processes
of the bird's brain, telling him of his hunger after his
long flight from southern Mexico; his ability to drink;
my stealthy movement on tiptoe to look at him out
the window; the movement of my eyes, seeing; the
innermost thought forming in my brain; and the
memory being stored.

The building block for all these movements
is omega-3 fatty acid, which we see advertised
everywhere nowadays. Omega-3 does not have the
usual square shape of a building block. It is shaped
like a bullet, a perfect missile sculpted for molecular
movement. This little missile fires itself by electrical
transmission, the way the message of electricity

moves along a telephone line, from the sender to the receiver. Messages are necessary in the body. The cells of the arm need to communicate with the cells of the brain. Even within the organ of the heart, each myocardial cell needs to connect with its neighbouring myocardial cell to keep the beat moving.

Omega-3 wires the body, connecting the brain to itself and to the rest of the body in the neural pathways, insulated by a myelin sheath, which surrounds the nerve fibres. Omega-3 also wallpapers the membranes of the retina to form the visual images translated and transported by the optic nerve into the brain.

On an ordinary day omega-3, gleaned from your daily diet, is stored in the liver. Strictly speaking there are three omega fatty acids—oleic, linoleic and linolenic—that are essential to the diet. Linolenic acid is probably the most valuable of all three and also the most rare.

All three fatty acids are the building blocks that maintain and manufacture crucial biochemicals in the liver for the body. They mastermind the health of the body. Their full story is still the subject of research and will be for a long time.

Life with very little omega-3 changes the chemistry of the brain itself, resulting in attention deficit disorder, depression, bipolar disorder, memory loss, schizophrenia, even suicide . . .

So eat foods rich in omega-3s, those of the old-fashioned kind: whole wheat breads with flax or enriched with the endosperm of seeds, such as wheat germ; legumes such as soya beans and peanuts; corn and sunflower seeds as well as poppy seeds; lamb and saltwater fish, especially mackerel and all sardines; most nuts, including hickories and walnuts; olive oil and nut oils; and eggs laid by happy hens that have been enjoying fresh air and wallops of sunshine. Nature's best, in other words.

Nuclear Cleanup

Eating watercress reduces nuclear contamination in the body...

The world is in a Catch-22 situation. We need clean, cheap energy. Many countries across the globe are looking to nuclear power as one solution.

A nuclear reactor uses the energy produced by burning highly reactive, naturally occurring metals such as uranium and plutonium. A flood of energy, called a chain reaction, is rapidly released. Controlling that reaction is like trying to contain a super-large firework in a box. The box must be strong and properly designed. It must be placed in a location that does not experience ground disturbances like earthquakes.

Something can go wrong quite easily, not so much because the chain reaction itself cannot be contained, but because human error comes into play. Once, a raccoon got into a North American nuclear station (they are good climbers) and caused a problem.

Another time, a candle caused a fire. The world was lucky that time. But Japan placed a reactor in a coastal area that received an oversized wave, and the backup systems failed. Canada has old pumping systems in one reactor. Money is often tight in these times of fiscal restraint. New parts are expensive. The damaging effects of radiation on concrete structures is still under study. The long-term problems of the materials from which these structures are built are not known, so decisions must be made with care.

When leaks or accidents happen at a nuclear facility, a reaction product called radioactive iodine is released into the atmosphere. This high-energy iodine is toxic to the human body, especially to children. Radioactive iodine interferes with the natural iodine of the body. Iodine metabolism is organized by a master organ called the thyroid, just under the chin to the front of the neck. The thyroid is a storage system for iodine. The iodine is metered out very carefully in a transit hormone called thyroxine, which, in turn, is regulated by the pituitary hormone. Thyroxine oversees the stability of a functioning body, young or old. When this hormone fails, things go seriously wrong.

Luckily there is a way to protect the thyroid: watercress, once a staple item of people all over the world. It's a plant that lives and thrives in water, which has to be absolutely clean and, if possible, flowing. Watercress is fussy about the water quality of its habitat. With clean water it will spread and grow into sheets of green food.

Watercress, *Nasturtium officinale*, is a member of the cabbage family and is an aquatic perennial. It can be found free-floating in water but more often holding on to the mud with its snow-white root system. The flowers are very small and white, occurring in the summer. The best time to pick watercress is just before the plant flowers; then you get its full, pungent flavour.

Watercress contains many of the vitamins and minerals important for the body, including calcium, iron and iodine. Long considered to be a medicinal plant, it acts as a stimulant like tea, coffee or chocolate. It is a diuretic, sweeping the kidneys clean. But it is for its iodine that the plant is now so useful, since many parts of the world are deficient in naturally occurring iodine, which protects the thyroid. Not only does a healthy thyroid boost vitality, it somehow reduces the crippling effects of allergies, one of the homoeostatic effects of thyroxine on the body.

Iodine from the humble pastoral plant watercress will help to dilute the radioactive version accidentally spilled from nuclear reactors into the atmosphere or sea, and absorbed by the human body. In science this process is called the dilution effect. Eating watercress will reduce the damage of the radioactivity and lessen its burden on the body.

Simplicity can sometimes be served up as delicious watercress soup.

Breastfeeding

A baby's health is laid down with essential fat . . .

The three of us were staring at the fish counter in our local supermarket. Christian and I knew exactly what we wanted: fish that was caught in the wild and brought to the store as fresh as possible. We also knew what we did not want: Canadian fish that had been caught off the continental shelf of the east coast and brought by trawler to China where the flesh was processed and saturated in some sort of preservative solution and transported back to Canadian customers as fresh.

The third person was a young woman, standing close to the counter and intently examining what was on sale. She seemed worried, uncertain, and did not know what to buy.

"Buy the halibut," I whispered to her. "It has not been cage grown. It is a deep-sea fish and it has not been re-frozen. It's your best choice for dinner tonight." When she smiled at me, I realized she was Emma, one of my daughter's friends. She confided, "I'm breastfeeding. My baby is just three weeks old. I want to eat only what is best for her. I know that fish is good for both of us."

What Emma was looking for is the Holy Grail for health, a crucial nutrient for her young baby to build a brain, nervous tissue, and lifelong wellness. The nutrient is one that I have had an interest in for some fifty years, ever since I learned of its significance while studying medical biochemistry, the omega-3 essential fatty acid called linolenic acid.

The reason biochemists call it "essential" is that a healthy body cannot be built without it. The fat molecule is a chain of carbon with an acid structure as an ending. For all the world it looks like a necklace with the acid acting as a clasp. This is what the acid does, too: it clasps onto various parts of the cell to operate. The necklace shape helps it to slink about, doing things that fatter, chunkier molecules simply cannot manage.

The two other essential fatty acids, oleic and linoleic, also look like necklaces, and have acidic endings that help them to grasp onto other things.

Every functioning organ of the body—the brain, the heart, the liver, the kidneys—and the neural pathways of communication must have a supply of these three essential fatty acids. But they cannot be made by the human body and must be eaten in food. Omega-3 fatty acids are found in fatty fish like sardines, herrings, mackerel, salmon, halibut and rainbow trout. These growing fish travel the oceans in shoals. On these travels the fish graze like cattle on the phytoplankton of the saltwater columns. They visit many species of cyanophyta plant organisms in the sea, and eat only those that contain alpha-linolenic fatty acid. This fatty acid is manufactured in each species of cyanophyta with a primitive thylakoid membrane, using a unit of the sun's energy, a photon. The fish get fat so they can survive the rigours of the migrations they undergo as part of their life cycle.

The other source of omega-3 fatty acids is nuts. Once upon a time the nut trees of the global forests had an astounding supply of nut flesh. To a botanist these nuts were fascinating in their volume, shape, size and form, a real biodiversity that is rapidly disappearing.

Even a hundred years ago, the hunter-gatherer ate one molecule of omega-3 fatty acid from nuts for every molecule of omega-6 fatty acid now found in the modern diet of meat, eggs and vegetables, according to Dr. Richard Béliveau, director of the Molecular Medicine Laboratory at UQAM—Sainte-Justine Hospital in Montreal. Now the balance has been tipped to one molecule of omega-3 fatty acids for every twenty of the omega-6 fatty acids. This dietary shift is leading us down the rocky road to cancer and to cardiovascular diseases.

No wonder Emma was staring at the fish counter. Her deepest instinct was to feed her child. It is the strongest instinct of all, that of a mother. But the cupboard was bare of omega-3 fatty acids. Society and science have failed that baby . . . have failed that child.

Mothers like Emma will have to pay more heed to the overfishing of our great seas. She will have to learn about the damage done to the sea floor by dragnets. She will have to demand that sanctuaries be established in the oceans to conserve fish stocks for future generations to ensure a source of these important foods.

SMALL FRUITS

Eat more small fruits every day . . .

Wild strawberries, tiny and delicious, are the first fruits I remember picking. The red berries were cheeky, tempting me from behind some green pennyroyal leaves and tiny ferns. But when I spotted them, they were mine. First I gathered them in my hand as I walked down the little *botharín*, the roadway to the farmhouse of my childhood. Then ambition pass-handled greed. I got a cup from the house and filled it to the brim.

My great-aunt was so impressed with my picking she led me into the cream room of the dairy, where huge wooden tubs sweated with the moisture of fresh cream waiting to be churned. She carefully poured a ladle of cream over the strawberries in my cup. I was let loose, carrying the cup now in both hands, back down the *botharín* to eat in peace. I sat on a mossy stone under the flame flowers of a fuchsia hedge. My memory is still etched with that pleasure.

Small fruits are important. Historically, throughout the ages of the human family, they have been collected, stored and eaten. The Haida nation of Haida Gwaii of western Canada kept them in large cedar bentwood boxes sealed with fat; the east coast nations mixed them into pemmican, a trail food; and the rest of the world either dried them in the sun or stored them in wine vinegars. Botanically, small fruits have their own family tribe on each continent. They all share common advertising ploys: eye-catching colours, fragrance and a tempting taste. The small fruit carries an extraordinary biochemical reward that is invisible and passes hidden in the taste. That reward for succumbing to temptation is not just health, but protection on a cellular level.

Fresh small fruits in season, such as strawberries, raspberries, blackberries, blueberries, cranberries, and black, red and white currants, all carry a botanical call from the wild. This call is ruthless and it is biochemical in origin: to reproduce. The little wild strawberry issues a flash of colour and fragrance so that it is eaten by either human or beast. Sieved through a fine digestive tract, its seeds are deposited in a nitrogen-rich medium, far from the mother plant, where it can begin a new cycle. Over time, the strawberry plant has learned to reward the picker so that he or she keeps coming back to the patch, year after year.

In exchange, the small fruit gives us a remarkable substance called ellagic acid. It was first isolated from eucalyptus trees in Australia in 1963. Then some Japanese scientists had a look at it and found that ellagic acid molecules could join together and form a chemical meshwork like chicken wire. This meshwork had fantastic detergent abilities in the cell, one of which was to reduce the mutagenicity of toxins coming into the cell and destroy their ability to initiate cancer. Since then, many laboratories have been working at breakneck speed, notably the Molecular Medicine Laboratory of Dr. Béliveau in Montreal and Professor Stewart Cameron's lab at the University of New Brunswick.

The person or animal who reaps the reward of ellagic acid receives enormous health benefits. In other words the DNA machinery of the plant rewards the DNA machinery of the person with something that benefits both in the end. To me this makes all small fruits a perfect medicine.

Take a look at just the cranberry family, so useful to the health of women. The mountain cranberry, *Vaccinium vitis-idaea,* is universally loved in Europe and Asia where it is called lingonberry. It is harvested in the late fall after a frost, which gives this berry its famed sour-sweet taste. It is eaten raw, canned, or cooked into jam or jelly. The jam uses the whole fruit. It is traditionally eaten in Europe as a condiment with meat or fish, or alone on bread. The Chipewyan nation of northern Canada also put this berry into pemmican.

The bog cranberry, *V. oxycoccos*, is the small fruit that is packaged either raw or frozen and found in our supermarkets. This berry is juiced and sold as straight cranberry juice or added to other fruit juices like apple juice to make a cranberry cocktail. The bog cranberry is found in Iceland and Eurasia, but it has made its mark in Canada. In the past at harvest time on the east coast of Canada the settlers would hold a cranberry festival. Scouts were sent out to inspect the berry's state of ripeness. A day was set aside for whole communities to harvest the cranberries—a health food that got them through the roughest of winters.

Many women become prone to urinary tract infections when stressed and overtired. Both species of cranberry, the mountain and the bog cranberry, can be used to keep such infections at bay. These cranberries carry two important biochemicals, arbutin and proanthocyanidin, which is related to ellagic acid. The arbutin is produced because the cranberry is a member of the heath or heather family. Arbutin is a urinary tract antiseptic. The relative of ellagic acid, proanthocyanidin, prevents the adhesion of E. coli bacteria to the skin surfaces of the urinary tract. This action is aided and abetted by a simple sugar, fructose, which appears when the frost has touched the cranberry.

Cloudberry, *Rubus chamaemorus*, another small fruit, also benefits the lives of women. It is a species of the circumpolar High Arctic of Canada, with a flavour that edges close to that of mango. It is still a favourite fruit of the Inuit, who preserve it in seal oil and occasionally smoke the leaves as a tobacco substitute. They also once used a root and stem decoction to treat barrenness in women. Science has learned that the ellagic acids in the plant can act as building blocks for reproductive hormones.

The scientific story of ellagic acid is rapidly evolving, but what is clear is that to maintain a modicum of health, small fruits should be eaten every day.

There are cultivars of strawberries, raspberries, blackberries and blueberries for all seasons. It is not such a bad thing to force yourself to get a cup and fill it with strawberries, then add a little creamed yogurt and sugar. Then sit behind your sofa in silence and eat. Nobody will know what you are doing . . . except the cat.

Zinger Ginger

Try a cup of ginger tea for a change . . .

Wild ginger is one of the oldest medicinal herbs in North America. Once upon a time wild ginger carpeted the virgin forest floor with its aromatic roots meeting the mosses at the stemline of trees. The medicine men of every first nation of Canada used ginger. In the spring, all of the aboriginal children were taught to recognize its peculiar, furry, kidney-shaped leaves and brownish-red flowers. This little plant still can be found hugging the ground, enjoying the rich humus of the deciduous forests.

The roots of wild ginger, *Asarum canadense,* were used to treat children and adults for colds, fevers and convulsions. They were used for headaches, especially long-lasting ones. A ginger root wash was used as a skin-surface antiseptic, sealing the skin against contact diseases. The medicine men used ginger as a physic, especially for older people, to strengthen their immune system and as a form of stimulant in the spring. They used a decoction of the mashed stems as a biochemical synergist to increase the efficacy of all the other medicines they were using. No organic chemist or medical biochemist has studied the polyphenols in wild ginger, a plant that is now becoming increasingly rare.

In the meantime, another ginger, *Zingiber officinale*, has been a medicinal herb in the Old World for thousands of years. It was beloved by the Arabs and used in India. The ancient Greeks imported it for its medicine. The Spanish brought it in from Jamaica early in the sixteenth century. To the Chinese, ginger was and still remains a very important medicine. Green ginger in syrup has been a delicacy in China for over five hundred years. This kind of ginger is also used as a general tonic or stimulant in the Middle East and Asia.

The roots of *Zingiber officinale*, beige-coloured and flattish, are to be found in every supermarket. The root grows as a mat, spreading quickly along the ground, needing the heat and the sun of the tropics. The green, upright stems and lance-like leaves feed the roots with extra moisture, condensed from the humid air. As a result the surface roots grow more readily, creeping along the ground. These roots, when they have thickened, are harvested. Then they are air-dried and boxed for the international market.

The cook also uses the medicinal ginger root. This is true for the wild ginger, *Asarum canadense*, and the cultivated, eastern ginger, *Zingiber officinale*. The root, minced or grated into food, is used as an herb for flavouring dishes. It can also be peeled and shaved into the dish to add a much stronger and dominant taste. This taste carries some heat with it, much like an Indian curry. Ginger can be pickled and served with sushi, added to carbonated water as ginger beer, and candied for sweet confections.

In my home, my husband and I eat candied ginger as a snack. We chop it up into little pieces. Then we add fresh nuts or raisins to the mixture. Sometimes we throw in some dark chocolate. I, of course, pick out the ginger pieces from under my husband's nose.

The biochemistry of ginger is very complex. The hot, pungent taste comes from gingerols and shogaols. The root also contains starches, proteins, fats, oils and an oleoresin. In this mixture there is also curcumin, the biochemical responsible for the flavouring of turmeric, *Curcuma longa*. The ginger root is packed with phenols. My own research shows the phenols of ginger are unlike any others because they are strongly bioluminescent under the beam of a scanning electron microscope.

I live in hope that a medical research team somewhere will choose wild ginger, *Asarum canadense*, as a topic worthy of investigation before it becomes extinct.

Industrial Food

Don't eat it on a daily basis . . .

The face of farming has changed all over the world during the past fifty years. The family farmer who once had intense knowledge of the seasons has silently evolved into a corporate, global giant of faceless names and nameless faces.

Our food is now an industrial product. This product is vertically integrated to include the production and sales of seed, fertilizer, herbicides, pesticides and agricultural equipment, tied together with a government lobby whose benefits are completely invisible. The corporation is on the move again, for transportation, processing, sale, advertising and the guarded distribution of the food products internationally. Vast tracts of prime, arable lands are changing hands across the globe, with an ultimate goal of corporate ownership. Governments are in the know and do not seem to care.

Our new industrial food is presented to us in an almost endless variation of pleasing products. But inside the boxes or bags there are only eight crops: wheat, rice, maize, potatoes, barley, cassava, sweet potatoes and soya beans. All others are not part of the gig.

This industrial food is born in a laboratory, where the plants' genes are torn apart, modified, reassembled and then carefully patented. The newborn seeds are grown with a succession of chemicals, first treated with fungicides and bagged for sale, then bathed in herbicides to beat down competition. Once the plants emerge they are treated with additional fungicides, followed by more herbicides and insecticides. The final insult for a field of mature potatoes is the "knock-down" chemical to kill off the top green growth so that mechanical harvesting can start. Before it sees market, the harvested spud gets a good dousing of chemicals to prevent it from sprouting. Then the spud hits the factory floor for sorting and bagging before it lands on the plate as food.

The three ugly sisters—salt, sugars and trans fats—are added to the mix. They press the buttons of the hypothalamus in the arena of desire: the craze to eat begins. One spoon or one slice or one bowl is never enough. It is not greed; it is the more powerful sibling of greed: the endorphin lust for food fired by the three ugly sisters, either alone or together.

Now and again, fear rattles the cage. The media pronounces that the world is running out of food because of shortages somewhere in this new global community of farming. There are latent whispers that water shortages are next.

The world is not running out of food or water. There is enough for everyone. The world is running out of wisdom. We have not learned to share our natural resources.

Food is a precious product of the natural world. And the human family has been dependent on it for millions of years. Both have evolved to be dependent on the other in ways that science does not completely understand. Good food made up of primary protein, sugars, fats, vitamins, phytochemicals and minerals is the only foundation of good health. And good health is, in turn, the only foundation of a thriving civilization.

Industrial food hoodwinks the body into believing a lie, for the three ugly sisters know all the tricks of the trade. Trans fats cannot be completely broken down in the human cell. Enzymes cut fats up into two carbon fragments until they are broken down for energy in a process called beta-oxidation. The trans fats leave one carbon fragment behind, and the cell does not know what to do with it. This carbon clipping gets put aside, somewhere, anywhere, and waits and accumulates.

Artificial sugars must be broken down, too, like all other foods. The Krebs tricarboxylic acid cycle is the main machine. A three-carbon sugar is put on the wheel and spun down to raw energy for the cell's mitochondria. But the sugar is in the wrong form. It presses the button in the brain for all sugars and nothing happens. The artificial sugar keeps pressing the button and standing at the door. This is the beginning of addictive behaviour, as you consume more and more of the artificial sugar and your craving is still there.

Salt does something else. It is made up of the mineral sodium married to a fast-acting hellion, a halide called chlorine. This table salt comes into the body in very large amounts and sets up the alarm everywhere. Sodium chloride is an osmotic agent, driving water from one place to another, from cell to cell, from organ to organ. It changes the blood. The volume increases as water pours into the blood itself, and the heart now has a heavier load, beating and forcing this extra volume all around the body. The heart and kidneys become exhausted, too.

Sodium from sodium chloride must be eliminated through the kidneys. It goes into the plumbing system there for filtration into urine. This process needs phosphate to keep everything in balance in the kidney itself. But the salty food has no phosphate travelling with it. And the kidneys become damaged. Much like the heart, they simply cannot do the work required of them.

In the body, there is a silent witness to all of this, an accounting system called epigenetics. The genome or DNA of each cell has a memory record in it. The tabs are called methylation. These are laid down forever, change coming only with a change of behaviour, which might shift the tabs again.

Like Snow White, the human family is in a deep sleep. We slumber amidst the rising tide of epidemics of obesity and cancer. We do not see what is happening around us because our eyes are closed. One day soon we will awake to see the curse of the corporation and realize that industrial food is toxic. Just like the cigarette.

BUSH FOOD

Nature holds hidden health . . .

A number of years ago I addressed the Assembly of First Nations. Afterward, a Cree chief made an observation to me about the health of his people, a comment repeated by his medicine man. I gave the comment a great deal of thought. Both men were from the boreal forest of Canada. The boreal is the circumpolar forest system in the north of the planet, which sits on the dome of the earth like a monk's tonsure. It is the last great forest. It is also the last great living tapestry of nature.

The Cree chief and his medicine man had noticed that as their people moved away from eating their native foods, they lost their health. First they became overweight and diabetic. Their teeth rotted or fell out. Then they developed cancers and heart problems followed by aging diseases they had never experienced before.

The peoples of the Cree Nation have a special name for food obtained from the wild on a seasonal basis, which has been on their menu for millennia: bush food. Bush food includes red meat from game, white meat from birds, fish from the rivers and lakes, vegetable protein from hazelnuts, the cambium of trees, aquatic plants and other plant protein, and the trail food snacks of dried fruit crushed into cakes and eaten with pemmican.

It so happens that bush food is an extraordinary form of nourishment. The red meat of deer, reindeer and caribou is not heavy with fat because the animals have been ranging in the wild and have walked or run off any excess fat they might carry. The meat is lean and filled with flavour from the wild herbs the animals have eaten over the course of their lives. The muscle texture of the meat is excellent for cooking, either stewing or roasting, and will hold together in the pot.

The white flesh of game birds does not carry a load of toxins because they have been hatched and raised in the nursery of nature by their mothers. These game chicks did not receive rations of veterinary-grade antibiotics. They do not suffer from growth spurts from food additives even before they can spread out their chicklet wings or grow pinfeathers on their breasts.

Fishes caught from the northern rivers and lakes of Canada are generally quite clean with the exception of those taken from waters contaminated by the runoff and wastewater from our numerous oil extraction, mining and milling operations. The scales on the backs of the fishes are intact. They are still healthy with a sheen that can only be obtained from oxygenated fresh water. These waters are cleaned by the natural chemical complexes produced by the willows and poplars that grow in these wet riparian places.

The vegetable protein from hazelnuts and from other edible nuts like the acorn and the walnut has a special formula for health. The tree packages primary protein into a shell, removing water in order to squeeze all that is best in nature into one little space. This is high-energy protein. Plant proteins hold more biochemical diversity than animal proteins. They carry the antioxidants that repair damage in the human cell. Many of these special plant proteins come from a wild origin like onions, *Allium drummondii*, and wild chives, *A. schoenoprasum*, which are laced with health-giving, sulphur-bridging abilities. The common cattail, *Typha latifolia*, provides starches and flour that have fed North American aboriginal peoples throughout the ages. Red samphire, *Salicornia rubra*, provides salt for cooking and flavonoids that mop up cellular toxins. The evening primrose family, *Onagraceae,* is a prodigious producer of B vitamins and anti-inflammatory compounds, all good for the body. The young leaves and stems are eaten like lettuce.

The small fruit the Cree consume are berries whose taste is unknown to urban populations. There is the cloudberry, *Rubus chamaemorus*. It is an herbaceous perennial with a golden-yellow raspberry fruit that offers an exotic flavour. In the northern world of the High Arctic this fruit is cherished for that unique flavour of a mild mango when eaten fresh or cooked with sugar. The delicious bog cranberry, *Vaccinium oxycoccos,* and the mountain cranberry, *V. vitis-idaea*, are also taken seriously as a food in Iceland, Greenland and northern Eurasia. These cranberries are picked and eaten as a medicine because they are high in fructose. This sugar, when eaten, repels E. coli bacteria in the urinary tract and forces them to leave by flushing them out and preventing a urinary tract infection.

All of the northern small fruits have one thing in common with the other fruit from nature: a clever mixture of complex, sweet sugars inside a coloured package. The skins carry a biochemical called ursolic acid. This powerful emulsifier or mixing compound helps in the digestion of foods and keeps the intestine healthy. The sugar polymers of northern bush fruit keep the body fit and free from fat by being an energizer, and by nursing the needs of the pancreas.

The nearest thing to bush food on the consumer shelf in the suburban world is organic food: free from chemical contamination, meat from animals raised free from stress, and fruit with its own coating of wild yeasts acting as a natural probiotic for the gut. Bush food is part of the wild brotherhood of organic food, free from internal molecular contamination, and it stamps a rose medallion of health firmly on both cheeks.

No Cell

How to use your cellular telephone . . .

A few years ago I was on a trip to Ireland where
I was collecting the unique germ plasm of an
ancient tree. I collected more than I bargained for,
the local flu. Being bed-bound in Sheen Falls' luxury
hotel did only one thing for me: it made me better.
I idled away the days being treated like royalty,
drinking fluids and trying to keep scrambled eggs
down, all cordon bleu. And served by a delightful
French waiter, no less.

Late one afternoon I received a phone call. Ireland
being Ireland, a good friend wanted to visit the sick
and maimed—me. So, he came for tea carrying the
wind off the Kerry Mountains with him in a gush.
This particular gentleman is a constitutional lawyer
beneath his pinstriped suit. He has a sharp brain and
is up to some judicial tricks that interest me greatly,
involving Ireland's ancient Brehon Laws, which

pre-date the waves of the Magna Carta and the Napoleonic Code he rides in his practice.

These laws represent the ancient jurisprudence of the Celts, a code laid down by the people of Ireland in the democracy of public discussion and decision, much like the laws of ancient Greece. They are being dusted off again. The Brehon Laws lay down ideas on copyright, environment and equality, and my friend holds the duster. Since all law is precedent based, I believe he will produce some golden nuggets in the due course of time.

He sat by my sickbed and we chatted about old times and our families. My young French waiter frisked about with a silver tray loaded to the hilt with afternoon tea, which he placed on a nutwood table looking out toward the falls and the grove of witch hazels that were dangling their golden blooms. Of course, appropriately, my friend was expected to pour. There is a strict ritual of tea maintained in Ireland, a soupçon of the past that is now more like a comfort food. My friend manned the large silver teapot, asking the correct questions about milk and sugar, when a telephone rang.

Immediately he put the Dublin silver teapot back

down on the tray. He stood up straight and shook himself a bit. Then he began groping in the right-hand pocket of his impeccable trousers, drawing on something that seemed to be very long. It kept coming and coming. I recognized something of the item. It was knitted: two plain, two purl. He kept pulling. As he pulled I could hear the ringing getting louder. Then suddenly it popped. The whole arrangement was in his hand.

(I forgot to mention that my friend is an eccentric. Ireland produces them in superior numbers. And everybody loves them, not so much for what they are but for what we all wish we could be.)

It was only in a split instant that I realized my friend kept his cellphone in a long knee sock made of untreated Aran-homespun wool. He turned the sock upside down and the phone slipped neatly into his open hand. He immediately held it as far away from his body as was possible. It was still ringing when he placed it near an ear. Slowly and carefully he answered. As he listened, his face broke into a sweat. When the conversation was over, he placed the phone back into its sock and returned it to its home in the right leg of his trousers. He whispered to me over the cups, "It's the rays! The rays!"

Maybe my friend's fear was excessive, maybe it was not; only time will tell. We know for sure that the effects of electromagnetic frequency (EMF) radiation are damaging. You have to hold the phone to your ear to listen, which means placing it next to the skull and brain. In adults the skull has thickened and the brain is relatively radiation immune. But in children the situation is different. A child's skull is thin and all of the biochemical pathways of the brain are in a form of rapid expansion. Children younger than eleven or twelve years old, whose brain banks and neural pathways are still growing into maturity, should use cellphones only in emergencies.

Carry your cellphone away from the body (not in your pocket). When speaking on these phones, switch ears constantly. Earphones reduce the risk. And keep your conversation short. Maybe some time in the future an EMF reflective barrier could be fitted into these phones, which would be easy and cheap to do. Such a retrofit was done on X-ray machines to protect the user from back-scattered rays. Yes, cellphones produce electromagnetic frequency radiation that is also absorbed by human soft tissue, the effects of which have not been quantified. While teams of scientists around the world are building a body of research on EMF radiation, we are all in a holding pattern, the babies, the children, the pregnant women, the teens and the rest of us. We wait to see and understand what exact dangers we all face.

And by the way, if you want to look really elegant, forget the Irish woollen sock cellphone holder!

Beggar's Buttons

Burdock is the new root vegetable . . .

Once upon a time, hedgerows, fencerows and forests were a common pharmacy with doors open to everyone. Knowledge of the use of wild plants was handed down from grandmother to grandchild, giving the child a survival kit for the future. Such interactions are dying out and we are all so very much the poorer for it.

One plant I carried in my young mind from such teaching has always been an interesting one to me because I was given the instruction about it in Irish. Later I asked questions about it in English. Then I added only a dash of the pepper of science, making it easier for me to swallow.

When I was small, I fell off a horse into a great swatch of nettles that stung my skinny little body. The nettles were mature and full of formic acid. In short order a series of red patches began to rise on my hands and face, arms and bare legs. The pain was like an inferno.

When I arrived back at the house, leading the horse, my great-aunt took a quick look at me. She wiped the flour off her hands and walked around the back of the house in silence. I followed. She stopped by a huge plant that grew near the dairy door and plucked off five large leaves. She carefully applied these leaves to my body, holding them by the edges. Then, using the heat of her hands through the leaves, she pressed on the worst stinging areas. She kept them there, applying mild pressure until the pain eased. Soon, very soon, I felt a whole lot better and gave her a big hug.

My darling great-aunt carried an encyclopedia of Druidic knowledge in her head. The plant she had carefully left growing by the dairy door was an old Celtic cure, burdock, *Arctium lappa*, a member of the daisy family and native to Europe and Asia. Early settlers brought it as a medicinal plant to North America. Burdock has many common names: gypsy's rhubarb, pig's rhubarb, snake's rhubarb, great burdock, edible burdock, cuckold and harlock. My favourite name is beggar's buttons because as a child I invariably came into the house with an extra set of brown, furry buttons or burrs clinging to my clothes. This of course is the clever dispersal mechanism of this wily plant.

The burdock has been naturalized in North America for a very long time. The aboriginal peoples have added it to their great pharmacopeia of plant medicines. Natives used burdock for bee stings and nettle rash, amongst other ailments. It is commonly used to relieve strained tendons in horse's legs after they have been ridden too hard, applied gently like a mild pressure bandage to the sore area. The leg is sponged afterward with warm water and then is towelled dry. Its effect is similar to the cooling gels that are now used in the horse world. Burdock was also used in magic where a doll was carved out of the root and used in ritual. The plant was an important source of pain relief, especially for strained backs, rheumatism and sore muscles. Three large leaves applied mildly bruised and warmed were big enough to cover the back. The bruising of the leaf releases its volatile chemicals and the heat helps the chemicals enter into the body for pain relief. It can similarly be used for headaches and earaches, applied as a loose-fitting bandage.

Burdock is a biennial, which means that it establishes itself in the first year from a seed germinated in the early spring and grows into the second year to flower and set seed for another cycle of growth. In the first year the plant creates the bulk and strength to carry it over into the second season in which it creates flowers and seed, a very expensive thing for a plant to do. Burdocks like sandy soil. The plant can grow up to 3 metres (10 feet) and the leaves can be 30 centimetres (1 foot) across. The best leaves for medicine are found lower down on the plant: they have more surface glands holding medicinal oils. Leaves from both one- and two-year-old plants may be used.

The burdock flower is produced in early summer. It is pink and like a small rosebud. This flower turns brown as it matures and curls into an extraordinary ball of burrs that catch on anything with cloth or fur. They are difficult to remove because of their tiny hooks. The plant uses this clever strategy to disperse the new crop of seeds. And this is the even more clever and money-making strategy of a modern product called Velcro, the inventor of which adapted the idea of the burdock's burr to replace buttons and zippers, and to mint a fortune.

Burdock is also a root vegetable. It is harvested at the end of the plant's first year of growth. The taproot, like a parsnip, can reach almost a metre (3 feet) in length if the soil depth allows. It ends in a fine taper, again like the parsnip. You cook the thicker portion of the white root, which contains inulin sugars, volatile oils, a lignan called arctiin, resin, several antibiotic chemicals and a bitter complex that needs further scientific work to characterize. Burdock root contains the same biochemicals as in the leaves, only in higher concentrations, and is used as a medicinal food all over the world.

Eating burdock root increases your resistance to infection. This resistance is conveyed through the lignan, arctiin, which is now being clinically evaluated for its potential to protect the body from cancers. The complex sugar, inulin, replaces starch as a sugar reserve and is also called alant starch, and is anti-diabetic, similar to the healthy sugars in the tubers of Jerusalem artichokes. Inulin as a carbohydrate is a health food for the body.

Harvest the first-year root of burdock as a root vegetable late in the fall, just before the first killing frost, to give the plant the opportunity to produce the thickest root. Like parsnips and carrots, it can be stored in sand in a root cellar for winter use for soups and stews. In addition, the second-year plant can be harvested for its leaf stalks, called petioles. These are the long attachment strings from the plant to the leaf blade. They can be eaten raw in a salad or can be boiled and mashed as a vegetable. These leaf stalks can also be candied for cakes and desserts, like angelica, adding a touch of the exotic to them.

The Japanese have claimed burdock as their own, calling it *gobu*. Years of breeding have produced root vegetables that are favourites in Japanese cuisine. *Gobu* also carries an expressed genetic trait called hybrid vigour from seed selection, giving the nursery trade of Japan superior seeds; these are readily available in seed catalogues and are the best for the vegetable garden anywhere in the world.

The last time I tasted *gobu* it was really fabulous. A Japanese friend brought it as a dish to add to our Christmas feast. The burdock root was sliced very thinly and marinated in soya sauce and sesame seed oil. Then it was stir-fried. The inulin sugars caramelized down to a dark sweetness. I just loved it . . . the taste was heavenly.

Chasing Cures

Don't just look at the Amazon . . .

I will tell you a true story about my life as a scientist that almost didn't happen, not so long ago. It took all of my courage to make it happen for the simple reason that I am afraid of snakes. Yes, I should be older and wiser and I am ashamed to admit it, but it's true: the snakes nearly stopped me from going on one of the scientific adventures of a lifetime.

First, some context: I believe many cancer cures are out there, waiting to be discovered. On top of that, Western civilization is its own worst enemy. Our global diet is terrible; the diversity of our food habits has evolved from eating 85,000 different species of plant foods to eating principally only eight, so there is no way we are eating enough phytochemicals to shield our cells from irregularities that become cancerous.

Toxic pesticides are being used by the millions of

tonnes, ignoring the fact that the plant or animal genome that is being destroyed is identical to our own design. Particulate pollution from industry, construction and warfare is so fine that it can carry hitchhiking, toxic molecules directly into our lungs. Genetically modified animals and plants with warped DNA are being used as food and medicinal substitutes.

Society is in a state of stress, with little laughter and less meditation and prayer. Everyone is in a hurry to go nowhere. Nonetheless, I believe in the magnificence of the heart of the everyday person who can conjure the extraordinary out of the ordinary. An idea, presented with courage and conviction, can change the world.

I published my book *Arboretum America: A Philosophy of the Forest* in 2003. In this book I spoke about ellagic acid and marmesin being potent anti-cancer agents, and of the native varieties of trees that used to be common in North America that are high in these compounds. The organic chemists of the Atlantic Forestry Centre in Fredericton and the University of New Brunswick picked up on this research. Now there is a rare Canadian tree of the orange family growing in their greenhouses, the seeds of which

I supplied. This tree is called the wafer ash, *Ptelea trifoliata*. (The tree has nothing to do with the ash family, *Oleaceae*.) Its biochemistry is being studied for possible cancer cures.

The wafer ash is a member of the orange or *Rutaceae* family. Somehow this tree survived the last ice age on the North American continent. The trees must have backed themselves up against rock walls facing due south so that the black box effect of the sun kept them from freezing to death.

The aboriginal peoples of eastern North America gave another name to this orange tree: the sacred tree. It is a medicinal tree of such strength that they treated it with the reverence of a holy entity. (And, by the way, something that terribly annoys me: our scientific community as a whole does not take seriously aboriginal medicine men and women. Their powerful arena of oral knowledge is ignored. Their medicines are being lost. I'll come back to this in a later essay.)

I have been chasing the rare sister tree of the wafer ash or common hoptree, *Ptelea trifoliata*, for over twenty years. I have done phone-in shows in the United States to alert scientists and naturalists to the hunt.

Faculty and students at all of the universities, especially botanists at Harvard, have been on the lookout for this lost tree. I've even asked major landowners like Ted Turner to search his territory for it.

Then, two years ago, I was down in Texas to give a lecture. I was asked to an early morning tea by a wonderful, wealthy Texan lady who has become my friend. I very nearly didn't go due to an embarrassing situation that happened the night before. I was bedded down in a huge, high, four-poster bed with a set of antique steps. During the night I forgot the steps and landed in a knot. One or two colourful words may have floated from my lips. So, therefore, I wanted to hide.

The long and the short of it was that the Texan lady knew my name. Another notable black sheep, a relative, Lord Delaval James de la Poer Beresford, had owned a ranch in the past next to her family's land in west Texas and New Mexico. I became excited because I knew the exacting habitat that my tree required. I asked if there were low elevations of mountains. She said yes. I asked if her ranch had ever been clear-cut. She said no. I held my breath.

This past March I returned to Texas. We flew to her ranch in west Texas. I was fitted out with a pair of heavy trousers up to my waist to protect me from snakebites, and hitched into a helicopter with the aid of the pilot. I climbed into a leather harness so I could be suspended out the open door. My earphones connected me to the sound system of the pilot so I could give him instructions. And I had a pair of powerful binoculars.

After days of gridding the rolling landscape and circling mountains and diving down into arroyos, I noticed something shimmering in the distance: yellow, round, silver dollar-shaped seeds laden with morning dew. The sight was unmistakable. It was my tree. It was growing out of a 7-metre (20-foot) depth of worked flint and arrowheads, surrounded by graves. The artifacts were seven thousand years old. It had been an ancient summer camping ground, a gathering place of the aboriginal peoples. I cried with relief. I knew that I had found a tree of great value to the world of science.

So immediately I set about taking cuttings and a few mature seed heads for planting. They have been left with the ranch's Mexican personnel with written instructions for growing. I am hoping to propagate this tree in the next few years.

The ancient medicine of this tree gives us another glimpse at how to tackle cancer research by making chemotherapeuticals that are a hundred times more effective through the use of synergistic biochemicals. Such chemicals are extremely rare in medicine, especially those from plant sources. This unique tree offers humans one of these synergists, which may potentially spare us the toxic effects of anti-cancer regimes.

The flora of North America is being ignored by universities, governments, corporations and private investors, as a rich source of medicine in favour of the flora of the tropics. The flash is not here. There is something else in the vegetation. It is a form of tenacity that defies all understanding. It presents life in the margins. It is only from the margins that real invention is squeezed, like water from a stone. The continent's medicine men knew this, less by instinct and more by knowledge. The sacred tree, *Ptelea trifoliata*, and its variants are nature's legacy to future generations. We should all give thanks for this gift, for this tree.

ABORIGINAL MEDICINE

There is much more to life than we understand . . .

The ancient Celts were a woodland people. They spread across Europe to Turkey. From their ranks they sifted out the gifted men and women, who were streamed into a pathway of learning that involved many disciplines—medicine, the environment, law and music. From their collective wisdom, the ordinary Celt understood very clearly that a human being was composed of the body, the mind and the spirit . . . the triad.

The triad philosophy is also common to most aboriginal nations of North America and to many others across the world. This thinking arises from the keen observation and in-depth knowledge that is accumulated by medicine men and women over their lifetimes. That knowledge is passed on to other generations to use in an oral manner.

The mind and the spirit have been generally

ignored in modern medicine. Both can be sick, either together or apart. The aboriginal world and the ancient Celts, through their studies, had medicines for the spirit and the mind, coming from local native trees.

The Celts and aboriginal healers alike treated extreme loneliness, or spiritual loss, a quality of the emptiness of the human spirit and an inability to smile at oneself, with the willow, *Salix*. There are many species and hybrids of willow in the global forest. They all carry a treasury of aerosol and water-soluble chemicals of different proportions that have become important modern medicines.

The diseases of mind and spirit in the North American aboriginal population were prevented or treated in sweat lodges through a special cleansing ritual. This purification of mind and spirit was also carried out by the ancient Celts in stone houses called perspiration houses or *Tig n'allais*. Local wood was burned to make an extremely hot fire that liberated antibiotic, fungicidal and antiviral chemicals from the wood into a closed space. These medical biochemicals worked synergistically for healing in a hot air mixture. The sick emerged from the sweat lodge or perspiration house whole again.

I believe that forests produce a tidal wave of medicines that ebb and flow with the seasons. They perform a vital scrubbing or detergent effect in the atmosphere, keeping it clean so that we can breathe the oxygen that the trees produce so efficiently. Forests are the vanguards of nature, standing in constant service, delivering a chemistry with which we are only now coming to grips. An example of that chemistry includes the taxanes used in the treatment of breast cancers. There are significant antivirals in the forests of Sarawak, the Malaysian tropical forests of Borneo, but those trees are, unfortunately, being cut today to manufacture paper pulp.

In the spring of last year I was asked to give a public talk in the open air of the South March Highlands in Kanata, Ontario. The question of forests came up. The South March Highlands, an 81-hectare (200-acre) piece of ancient woodland, was under threat within the boundaries of the city of Ottawa. It was up for grabs as a housing estate. The trees would come down, the box turtles would die. I had previously visited this forest by invitation and had written a scientific paper on the woodland itself and the astounding botanical importance of the trees that were harboured there, both rare and endangered species. In my presentation I said that I thought that greed would win this fight, and the South March Highlands would soon be gone.

After my talk, a gentleman from the Algonquin Nation came from the crowd and spoke to me. We discussed the importance of this ancient forest, which had been an island on the Champlain Sea and a sacred place for his people since time immemorial. He asked me if I knew or had been introduced to Grand Chief Commanda. No, I had not. But I was careful to ask this man to send a message to Grand Chief Commanda to ask for his prayers because I knew that my spirit needed strengthening to fight this kind of greed.

When I got home after the talk, Christian and I decided to have a barbecue. We would have some steaks and a glass of wine. The air was warm. There was absolutely no wind. The stillness around us gathered the smell of smoke and fire, which kept the mosquitoes and black flies away. We relaxed together, chatting and sipping wine. The sun had edged behind the catalpas, so it was thinking of setting. The sky had hit gold, in a claim that was spreading westwards down to the horizon. There was no reclamation, yet, of the night.

The charcoal grill was setting down its black lines on the meat with a lovely sizzle. We were both by now staring at the coals with a good hunger coming along to lead us to our evening meal. The wine, too, lulled us into a reverie. Then all of a sudden, the red pines to my left began to whip about sharply. We both looked up into their canopy, which was being flailed about by a tempest. It was strange because nothing else was moving other than those pine trees, despite the fact that there are plenty of other trees in this garden.

All of a sudden a bolus of energy seemed to embrace me, coming from the red pine trees. I was now attached to them in some way. We were one, together, in a unity of being. The wind continued but it centred on me and then went inside my mind as if led by an invisible hand placing something extra within my consciousness. The word "Commanda" flooded into me, washing through and energizing me. Then I knew what was happening. Commanda, who was the grand chief of the Algonquin peoples, was sending me his healing through long-distance medicine: ghost medicine.

Ghost medicine outlines the spirit and draws a boundary around it, rendering the largesse of your own spirit perfectly clear. There is an energy to it and a feeling of human warmth that arises from your whole being, like in gift-giving. Then after this first awareness, the additions take place, the presence of someone else standing within your spiritual territory. There is a feeling of homage to the abilities of that other human being who can travel into this space of the spirit. There comes a wholeness, too. You never thank the medicine man or woman for the gift of ghost medicine. It is simply not done; the spirit of the giving is too great.

I return, as always, to the Celtic triad of body, mind and spirit. They are the pillars that support the dimensions of life without which we would all be one-dimensional and only half-alive. Science and medicine have a long way to go.

I received news of Chief Commanda's death the following day. He had visited me in the form of ghost medicine on his way to meet his death and had died only minutes before that wind. Such visits are common in the Celtic culture, too. They are called *sí gaoithe* or spirit winds, when the body releases the spirit.

And that spirit was Commanda.

Slow Down

Relaxation is beneficial for health . . .

Nobody wants a headstone that reads, "I was dying to work twenty-four hours a day. Now I lie under six feet of sorrow." So get out there and enjoy yourself. Treasure the moment, for it is a moment of your own life.

When I want to relax I dive into a special place I hold in my mind on Prince Edward Island. This little, half-moon-shaped piece of land lies on the east coast of Canada, bracing itself against the full lash of the sea. My special place is on the north shore where a brook runs a racecourse over rich, red rocks to meet the salt of the sea.

I sit on one of those rocks. It is a perfect seat, flat, in the middle of the stream with all of its rushing and rippling sounds. My back is to the sharp "V" of the valley in the cliff through which the brook winds, sweet-scented with pink-faced Joe-Pye weed. I face out to the ocean with its wand of waves. The wind against me is always clean and has a drone to it, weary from the flight to reach land. Sand plovers appear on the brook's spreading ebb in a silent symphony of movement. They pick at some fragments of life from the sand and tide that only they can see. They rush together like a stringed instrument whose music is played on fragile, twig-like feet.

I sit still, fearful that my movement might cause a shift in any single thing at all. I listen to the sea. I feel it in my mouth and bones. I dream with the stream as the water rushes by. All of the tiny sounds of life move as an orchestra of scattered music around me. No note goes unnoticed in this gentle place of stones. And, then, if I am lucky, a great mammal of the sea rears up to suck air and spout water like some supernatural waterfall. Surprised, the hidden monarch butterflies rise from their feast on the nectar tables of Joe-Pye weed behind my back. They float over me like autumn leaves, brilliant with orange and red and black, enamelling the azure blue, windswept skies.

Now you know the place where my dreams begin. I go there to relax. It is my place. It will always be my place and mine alone. I turn on the feelings and sensations whenever I feel I need them. It is a place that will live as long as I am alive because it exists in the landscape of my mind.

My visit to paradise is the beginning of meditation. It is a form of prayer. The sweet sounds are the mantras of nature. These sounds are always soft and have a soothing effect. These sounds, too, are a religion in themselves because they beget peace and calm—the very opposite of anger and angst.

Relaxation and meditation are good for the soul. But the big surprise is that they are extremely important to the health of the body. Relaxation acts in a holistic manner. It starts with the brain and goes to all of the major organs, fine-tuning the entire human machine. Lowering stress reduces the flow of cortisol, the anti-inflammatory hormone produced by the adrenal cortex of the kidneys. It is like having a good, sound sleep without ever going to bed.

The central nervous system is the highway of the body that transports the messages of the brain in a command-and-obey fashion. Some of these commands are autonomous and outside of our control. But others are within our control through prayer and meditation. When we relax, the chatter of the day is released and the highway is cleared of traffic. Even the beating heart is affected by prayer and meditation. The pulse of each beat slows to a stronger, even keel, which gives the special, polarized muscle cells of the heart a change from their daily frantic race.

Rest, relaxation and meditation are good. Prayer is even better, carrying benefits that science cannot fully explain. They have always been there waiting for us. They are free. They are simple and easy.

Sit on my stone with me. It is large enough for both of us. But please don't speak. I just love the music of that silence.

Part II

HOME AND GARDEN

I n these essays on home and garden, I invite you
into my root cellar and show you around. This is
how I live. I grow a vegetable garden and store the
produce in the root cellar. Then I know exactly what is
on my plate. There is an immense satisfaction in that.

The kitchen is the hub of the house. Most of us
seem to spend a lot of time there. It is where food is
prepared and that is a magnet for us all. But there are
hazards in the kitchen. They are invisible and come
from human-made materials and fibres. Rectify
these hazards for the sake of your own health, and
the environment's, by choosing to use natural
products, especially in the kitchen. They are safest
in the long run.

My garden is my oasis. As I travel down the long
half-mile road through the woods to my garden I know
that I will see something beautiful in all seasons.

Returning to the garden is always a pleasure for me.
Every day I take time to enjoy it.

For everybody, the backyard or the balcony can be
a window into nature. Sometimes the tiny gardens
are the best, those whose summer fragrance drifts
out into the public pathways. Many schools and
institutions of North America have changed their
gardens into places of wonder, based on the bioplans
I've published in my book *A Garden for Life*.

You will find many good tips in this section to
help you when you are wearing your gardening
gloves. My garden is very large so I have to use a lot
of shortcuts and labour-saving thinking around
my flowers and trees.

One thing I like to do is to plant a flower or tree
that represents a friendship. Paul's tree is a weeping
willow given to us by the godfather of my daughter,
Erika. It is his little patch of property. Another is a
beautiful crimson maple, a wedding gift from Ray
and Joyce, two of our oldest friends. The local
coroner gave me violets.

And for heaven's sake buy some good Adirondack
chairs, ones with wide handrails that will hold a glass
of wine or a cup of tea. Plant them out in the middle

of your lawn, in some evening shade. They are an invitation to other gardeners, like a welcome mat.

One of my wooden chairs has had a porcupine munch on one of its legs. Another has had an owl perch on the back. A fisher was seen near another. Birds seem to think that I put them out only for them. Maybe they are right. But when I come out with my cup of tea, they had better make room for me!

Grocery List

A direct expression of modern living . . .

Everybody makes a grocery list. People who live alone and families alike may be caught with such a list deep in their pockets in the tangle of small change and car keys. Christian is a good example. You would never in a thousand years expect a man who has designed the gold standards for travel into space to know the price of food as it goes up or down. He does. And he keeps a wish list, too. It has something to do with welding projects.

Not so long ago the grocery list was a bucket. The farmer filled it with spuds or cabbages or apples. Plucked chickens went into one and maple syrup in another. The bucket, full of local food, was handed across the kitchen door. The grocery list now expresses not only what we cook for ourselves and our families (if we cook), but the story of global transportation. This is not the age of the spice trade.

This is the age of the bulk container food of the commodity market, expressed in enormous sums by the stock and commodities exchanges of the world.

The prices on the modern shopping list tell the story of cheap oil, which fuels cheap transportation. National food security is largely ignored and is exchanged for the poverty of imported labour. Farmers are forced into impossible situations to compete for sales. The soil is suffering. Fields are growing ever larger while their riches are being swept away into streams, rivers, lakes and oceans. Farm animals are turned into the slaves of the food trade, penned into tiny spaces. Slaughter ships are on the high seas outside the international limits and nobody exactly knows what goes on out there. The meat comes back limp, filled with liquid and the muscles threaded with adrenalin.

This disastrous behaviour is the target of aware consumers attempting to rewrite and re-order their grocery lists. People are making longer lists with notes after each item about provenance and health. They are buying much more carefully. They are thinking about price and what they can afford, but they are also thinking of something very different as they walk down the lanes of the grocery store with that white list in their hands. They are now thinking seriously of what the planet itself can afford.

Many people are now thinking of sustainability in a broader sense. Mr. and Mrs. Main Street of North America and Mr. and Mrs. High Street of Europe are making a shift in their choices of food, and much of it is good. Their revised lists are a new expression of their needs for the welfare of their own families and for the future of their children.

Grass-fed beef is now on many grocery lists. These animals have spent their lives in green pastures in which grasses and clovers have been growing. The animals have lived out their days, sleek with health, in the company of their own kind, in sunshine. Their meat is high in all of the D vitamins, and is healthier for the family. If the meat is from organically raised stock, so much the better.

Suddenly, free-range chicken is all the rage. This chicken, surprisingly, tastes like chicken and not like elastic rubber bands that have been boiled and bleached overnight in some swamp. Free-range chickens walk proudly, clucking to the sun and rain. They grow a sheen on their feathers like all other birds and come to the call of the cock for their protection. These birds, too, have extra vitamin D content in their flesh and in the skin, where the taste lies. Vitamin D protects them from the many viruses of the chicken world, which in turn helps to protect us from diseases.

Wild, line-caught, ocean fish, selectively harvested, are now available in many seaports on certain days of the week; shoppers rush to the boats in glee. This fish is fresh. It does not taste like the fish that has been caught by ocean-going trawlers with destructive dragnets, transported thousands of miles for packaging and refreshed in a chemical bath that helps to hold the form and structure of the flesh until it hits the cooking pot and then emerges as a glop that tastes like wood pulp and glue with an antibiotic sauce. Fresh, line-caught fish once again grace our tables as the wholesome food nature intended.

Vegetables fare better on the new grocery list, too. We can now buy organically grown potatoes from a local farmers' market, or in a separate section in the supermarket. These tubers have not been soused in fungicides and pickled in pesticides. The taste of the spud comes through with shocking surprise. They are good.

The same is true for the best of the veggie world; for carrots, summer turnips, beets, winter turnips, squash and all of the ranks and rows of other root vegetables that visit the soup pot in the kitchen. Garlic bulbs are increasingly showing their faces on counters, glowing with local health. They go onto the grocery list, too. And their faces are not painted with herbicides either.

Fruit flows gently onto the list. A lot of small fruit is locally produced. Increasingly this fruit does not rot overnight with the strange white bloom of mucor fungi caused by an overuse of systemic poisons. It is joyous and free. It will go down the colon, sharing the space and mingling with resident bacteria that pluck from the digested fruit all of the B vitamins to transport across the cell's causeway into the bloodstream. Calcium is liberated for work with the human hormone insulin to control the flow of sugar in the bloodstream, too.

Someone is twigging to the marketing of nuts. They are being packaged under vacuum with some nitrogen gas to keep the oleic fatty acids from going rancid.

The grocery list is changing. It's getting better and better. And people are too. Health is on the horizon, again. For us and for our planet.

HOME TIPS

H ere is some old-fashioned kitchen cunning from an Irish woman that will help with the bottom line and keep health in your home.

Ireland is full of moulds and mildews. Many houses are built from stone and heating is expensive. The Georgian house I lived in as a child seemed to smother me sometimes with the smell of mildew. Occasionally we had to keep an anthracite fire burning for a week in each room, not so much for its heat but to subdue the mildew.

Mildew has returned to haunt me again. This time all of North America is being fed the fumes. Climate change has done something nasty and it will probably get worse for us all. The carbon dioxide portion of the atmosphere is steadily on the increase; it steps up every year. This increase physically changes the chemistry of the atmosphere. Carbon dioxide, in the presence of humidity, turns into carbonic acid. Mildews and moulds love carbonic acid. It makes them thrive.

Mildews and moulds are fungi. They are classified botanically as plants, but in some ways they differ from plants and that makes them difficult. They reproduce by releasing spore babies, millions of them. Spores are as light as ash. They love humid, warm, acidic air rich in carbon dioxide. They ride this acidic wind right into your home and set up house under your nose.

Spores can land on clothes, on walls, on boots that are still damp inside, around toilet tanks, under sinks, in closets, on the soles of shoes in storage, on paper products in cabinets, on any athletic kit, on camping gear, and around the household plants. The dry spores settle in a damp place, any damp place. They begin to germinate much like a seed. Soon the growth spreads into a bloom like a mat, and the maturing mildew or mould is on its way to cause the entire household, including the pets, health problems with allergies and breathing difficulties. There are moulds that are so toxic that they put one's life in danger if you breathe them in; these need to be dealt with by professionals.

Airing is one answer. Clothes, bedclothes and all fabrics can be hung out on a clothesline in the direct sun for at least twenty-four hours. The airing dries out the fibres of the fabric and treats the mildew, mould and the spores to a dose of sunshine in which there are high-energy spectra that are toxic to moulds and mildews. If the infestation is bad, bring the items in from the dampness of the night air and hang them out again the next morning for another stretch, shaking them during the day to release the fungal debris.

The next item in the kitchen arsenal against mildew is very cheap: baking soda or sodium bicarbonate. This household product dissolves in water to make an alkaline wash. This wash destroys moulds and mildews, which cannot survive the high pH it produces in solution. This killing machine is non-toxic to all members of the household including the pets. A wash of one tablespoon per litre of warm water will do the trick for cleaning walls, floors, refrigerators or any item that has become mouldy.

Leave the bicarbonate wash to dry on its own and evaporate naturally. The moisture disappears into the air and leaves behind on the item a very fine microscopic film of bicarbonate salt, becoming a solid again, almost like a paint finish. This film prevents the airborne spores of mildews or moulds from growing on the surface spaces. It acts as a protective, non-toxic shield into the future. Did I mention the word "cheap"? It's cheap, also!

In the kitchen and bathroom I use two kinds of solid soap. One, a hand soap for washing my hands and face, contains rose oil that pays attention to the subsurface capillaries of the skin, keeping them healthy. The second is a rougher kind called washing soap. It is manufactured as a large yellow bar, about three times the size of hand soap. It is made from sodium oleate or sodium palmitate and caustic soda in the saponification process. This soap has excellent detergent or cleaning abilities. I use it for stain removal on clothes prior to washing. This takes just minutes and considerably reduces the amount of water needed in washing clothes. Reducing water consumption is important to the entire planet.

My home is in the country. As the days of summer draw to a close, the ants get moving for a new, dry, warm home. Swarms land on the roof and the invasion begins. We repel ant invasions with naturally occurring boric acid, placing a few drops on wax paper on the chemical trail used by the ants. The ants like the sweet taste of boric acid, carrying it back to the nest. A few days of exposure to this acid is sufficient to discourage these household pests. Boric acid occurs in nature as a mineral called sassolite. It is colourless and odourless on the wax paper, which we burn after it's done the job.

In areas with hard water, such as mine, toothbrushes don't last very long. The bristles become encased with calcium from the water, and become as stiff as metal. Sometimes these bristles poke and injure the gums and it may take up to a week for the gum to heal. Place the toothbrush into a solution of white household vinegar for a few hours. Work the bristles with your thumbs to dissolve and release the calcium. Rinse with warm water. The toothbrush bristles are soft and ready for action once again.

I store dry foods in glass, including a few grains of rice in flour and beans to keep them dry. I also take meat products out of plastic as soon as I bring them home and repackage them in waxed and brown paper, which I then wrap in plastic to prevent desiccation. This ritual buys an extra month in the life of the meat in the freezer and prevents the cross-contamination of odours from other foods.

I am very fussy about my cooking vessels. I like heavy steel, because it saves on the energy bill. A heavy pot will hold its heat long after the stove has been turned off, so slow cooking can continue if the meal is timed properly. Non-stick coatings on cooking vessels wear off in time, most often into the body with the meal. Some of these inert plastics can sit in the microstructures of the human cell. These plastics may possibly be a hazard to some people in the future, especially children who have the full run of their lives ahead of them. So it is better to be safe than sorry. Avoid non-stick coatings.

Using a dishwasher in the kitchen can have very unexpected health effects, especially if the kitchen itself contains cupboards and countertops made of artificial materials. Plastics seem to be chemically stable, but they are not. These materials are affected by light and aging, which cause the plastics to break down, slowly. Also, many plastics, even though they are made up of polymeric units stacked together and aligned into rows, have the ability to loosen a few of the polymer units. These become airborne and toxic in large amounts, as any firefighter knows. Many of these plastics, such as vinyls and phthalates, produce monomer or single-unit molecules that become airborne with the warm, hydrated air of dishwashers. These molecules contaminating the air can become an irritant for some members of the household, especially those with chemical sensitivities.

And as a passing thought, if you happen to see a neighbour's cat or dog leave a garden gift for you to clear up, scatter orange, lime, lemon or grapefruit peel about. Maybe even plant a biennial like the gorgeous tall meadow clary, *Salvia pratensis*, in your garden. It will reseed itself with glorious, grey, furry leaves and racemes of pretty pink flowers. Dogs and cats positively detest this sage. They will not go near it, let alone deposit a gift. So you can look your neighbour in the eye and smile. Again.

TIN HOUSE

Protect your home against electromagnetic fields . . .

Physics is one of my passions. I came upon this wonder early in my life and I have never let it go. Stephen Hawking and Einstein are my bedside companions, the knowledge of the workings of the world just a page away.

As a twelve-year-old, I attended a convent school. It was a private place for girls, set on an island in the River Lee. The nuns who taught were professionals who freely floated between the school and the local university. In this environment, for me, physics won hands down over domestic science.

Our first day in the science lab proved to be a terrifying one. As we bunched around the Bunsen burners and played with the flint igniters in a heavy smell of gas, we were told to settle down and read while Sister Mercedes was busy with paperwork. I read. Five minutes later, I told her I knew the chapter on hydrogen. She looked up and told me to go on to the next one. I did. Five minutes later I knew the chapter on oxygen. Then I made the big mistake of telling her that, too.

She glared at me. She threw down her gold writing pen on the desk in anger. Then she stood up. Still with her beady eyes on me and her fingers on her crucifix, she walked toward me. The other girls were, by now, crouching in absolute terror. They had stopped reading, all of them, turning into statues. The saint and the sinner had locked eyes. "Tell me," she hissed. "And shut the book."

So I began, first with the page number, then the position of the script on the pages and the title of the chapter in bold. I began to recite the properties of oxygen line for line. The images were in front of my eyes as if the book was open, but I could see something finer in my memory. I noticed the style of the book—it was a new one, fresh from the presses of an American university—so I described that, too. And the publisher's name and address. Sister Mercedes stood transfixed. Without one word she left the room and returned with the headmistress, a nun we called Bona. Both sisters stared at me.

I expected expulsion. I was by now almost fainting, because expulsion for me spelled only one word: "orphanage." I had to hold on to the desk to remain standing. I finished my recitation and they left, talking a mile a minute. Nobody uttered one more word to me about that incident, not the girls or the nuns. But I received an excellent education at their hands, because soon the nuns brought in the heavy guns, the professors from the university, to teach me.

In addition to this I had my bachelor uncle at home, a chemist who believed that his beloved niece needed to rub noses with his immense and diverse library of first editions. We would read poetry, plays, science and literature of an evening. And of course the riveting subject of physics constantly came up to entertain both of us. Later, when I did research for my PhD in the United States, my minor subject for my thesis was, "The Effects of Radiation on Biological Systems." I always went for the double whammy.

Biological systems like humans, animals and plants are fragile. They are only as strong as their weakest link, which is carbon in all of its glory. Carbon is an atom found everywhere. It is the richest element in nature, existing in living creatures and in the dead, in the sky, the earth and the oceans. Carbon is a four-armed atom, with the ability to hold four other atoms at the same time; the arms are called bonds. This is the design of life. It's simple and straightforward.

Carbon bonding has laid down life as we know it. This carbon has a past, a present and a future. In the far distant past, carbon flooded Earth's atmosphere in the form of carbon dioxide, making it toxic. Slowly this carbon fitted itself into molecules, big ones and little ones, clearing out the skies. The carbon molecules became plants, animals and humans. Then humans got busy releasing the carbon back into the skies. We don't know where it will go. The future for carbon is a return to the atmosphere as a gas, making it toxic for us once again.

In addition, we don't know everything about this carbon bonding business. New research is surprising us every year. There are forces of attraction within carbon, defining it as the essential component of living material. These forces always involve energy, no matter to which other atom the carbon atom is attached. This diversity within the world of molecules makes carbon a celebrity. The energy of bonding is still being scientifically defined.

In recent years, industry has begun generating enormous amounts of a "new" form of energy—electromagnetic fields (EMF)—through the proliferation of modern communications devices like cellphones and the now-ubiquitous wireless networks. This new energy is a fundamental physical force that is responsible for interactions between charged particles. EMF will have an effect on carbon bonding. The effect will vary depending on the structure of the molecule in which the carbon sits. An example would be a change in charge of the spiral form of DNA. Very few laboratories have looked at the effect of EMF radiation on biological systems.

Very little meaningful research has been done on the effects of EMF outside of the classified research of weaponry. One little piece of science by Dr. Gerd Oberfeld, physician and EMF researcher, and his team in Salzburg, Austria, show that EMF, particularly microwaves, change the proteins in cell membranes and flood the mitochondria, which is the powerhouse of the cell, with free electrons. This cascade of electrons could affect memory and learning.

Other research teams have shown teratogenic, or DNA-altering, effects in the embryos of mice and turtles. Plants have been shown to exhibit stress through the production of an excessive amount of the amino acid alanine, which means that there are some triggers altering the DNA of the plants.

Christian and I have designed our home to reflect some of the EMF from microwave and cellphone towers and created living spaces with reduced EMF levels. We lined the outside walls with reflective builders' foil under the wooden cladding. The interior finish is also backed by foil. This double layer of reflective material significantly reduces the EMF irradiation in the inside of the house. It is cheap and easily incorporated into the design of a home. At the very minimum, a baby's room should be protected.

There is no doubt in my mind that we will learn how to safely manage EMF. Until then, I will remain secure in my tinfoil home.

Root Cellar

The nearest thing to garden-fresh . . .

My root cellar is my private boudoir. It is my pride and joy. This room is not important for its looks, but for what it contains. And to me, it is a testimony to all my training in science because I use every bit of ingenuity I possess to grow my food organically and then store it away to be eaten during the dark months of winter and spring. My root cellar is my rough diamond cut from the treasure of my garden. And you will never taste a potato as good as one of my Magdalen blacks!

The root cellar is attached to the house, but a few steps away from my large country kitchen. The walls and roof are superinsulated. There are two aluminum air vents placed a foot from the ceiling for air circulation. Our well is set into the rough concrete floor of the cellar, an encased well with expensive bronze fittings, money wisely spent to keep the well water clean. The well also acts as a natural humidifier, keeping the food fresh. The root cellar can withstand outside temperatures of -40°C (-40°F). If the temperature goes below that reading for several days, one single candle set in a large tin on the floor keeps the root cellar at the required 2°C (35°F) to prevent freezing.

And while I am about it, I will admit to something else. I simply adore flowers and love to have them in my house every day of the year. My wealth is measured by paperwhite narcissi, not by my bank account. I pot up spring bulbs like the fragrant grape hyacinths, hyacinths, daffodils and various African amaryllis and take them out week by week to enjoy. They fill the house with their personae and various scents, helping me to look out at the snow and feel smug.

The first action in the yearly cycle of the root cellar is in August, when we scrub down the floors, bins and walls with a 2 percent chlorine bleach solution to sterilize them. We haul the wooden storage crates out to stand in the direct sun, turning them so every surface has a chance to bask. The ultraviolet light acts as a sterilizer, killing off all fungal spores and growth. This takes about a week. Because the climate has changed in North America to produce greater summer humidity, the root cellar is vented with fresh air or with a dehumidifier for a week or so until it is dry.

I dig our potatoes days after the foliage dies back. This is an elaborate process for me because I have a potato collection of rare and heritage species that I carry over from year to year. Some of these potatoes are not available commercially; they represent a genome that is very valuable to the future, a seed bank of sorts. There are early potatoes that are dug in mid-summer, and the more serious kind meant for winter storage are dug in the fall.

I dig each grouping of potato separately: the early, the mid-season and the late varieties. They are then air-cured on the fresh soil in the garden, spread out to catch the sun. They are rolled over at midday until every part of the potato skin is dry. They are cleaned by hand brushing. This curing process is important to the storage life of the potato. Each mature potato has a skin called a cortex. This cortex must be seared by about eight hours of sunshine to drive the potato into full-blown dormancy that will last the winter. Some of my potatoes, especially the Magdalen blacks, carry an unusual genetic trait. They hold a white layer that contains lectin biochemicals just underneath the cortex. Lectin is an important anti-cancer chemical found in some foods. I treat these potatoes like gold.

Following their sunbath, all the potatoes get a light dusting of dried wood ashes while they are still on the ground. I then line the storage boxes with saved newspapers, cleaner and cheaper than anything else. The potatoes are boxed, labelled, ashed a little again and wheeled into my boudoir, the root cellar, for winter.

Root vegetables, like carrots, beets, turnips, radishes and parsnips, all have varieties suited to winter storage, laced with more vitamins, anthocyanidin colours and potash salts than the early varieties. They are sweetened by cold weather, which prepares the vegetable for its winter life. The sugars in the root vegetable are changed, too, re-formed and packaged into polymers. Polymerized sugars are perfect for the pancreas, making insulin work longer, keeping blood sugars in a better balance.

Snapping the leafy tops off the root vegetables by hand leaves them in a perfect condition for storage. I select and Christian packs the best of the best vegetables, laying them down sideways in clean sand, one layer of vegetables followed by a 2.5-centimetre

(1-inch) layer of sand to separate them for winter and spring months. We put the carrots away first, then beets, turnips, and winter radishes. Parsnips are always last because the cold improves their flavour so much.

It always seems that the leeks are in a race with the gladioli. Dig leeks in November, two minutes before the snow or when you can see your breath condense in the crispy air. Shake them free of root soil and pack them upright in sand in pails, packed very closely together with just a little sand for separation. The leek tops get a 15-centimetre (6-inch) haircut and inspection for health. It is important for the outer skin to be intact. Like the onion, leeks contain alliin in all their cellular tissues, an anti-cancer chemical that stays in the stored leek into spring.

The gladioli are my summer cutting garden, the full 35-metre (100-foot) row of them. I breed them for their colours of flame, yellow and orange. Of course, more have been added over the years, including a very fine one this year, a tiger gladiolus complete with stripes. Lifting them, storing them to cure in drying sheds and finally cutting the corms into open boxes, is something I think I will never have time to get to, but I always do.

Cabbage, too, has many faces. There are white and red cabbages and a worried-looking form called Savoy cabbage. There are Chinese members of this family with elongated heads. These are harvested in the fall when the heads are firm, just before the killing frost. We place them in layers in clean wooden boxes for winter salads. Cut and collect cabbages for sauerkraut and kimchi immediately, while the sap content is still high. Sauerkraut and kimchis are fermented using the wild yeasts that grow on the cabbage. A little rock salt is added only to extract the plant juice in which the fermentation process proceeds. Sauerkraut and kimchi are health foods *par excellence*, containing phytochemicals called glucoinolates that protect the gut from cancers.

Store nuts like hazelnuts, black walnuts, butternuts, kingnuts, shagbark hickories and edible acorns on a layer of steel mesh so that the air can flow between them. Drying shrinks the flesh so the nutmeat is more easily released. Nut flesh contains ellagic acid, a cell-growth inhibitor, which stops the growth of cancer. The flesh meat of nuts is a primary, first-class protein laced with essential fats that protect nerve and brain tissue.

Oh yes! And then there are the quarts of garlic dills, tomatoes with basil leaves and bottled fruits. On other shelves I have jars of chutneys, relishes, sauces and jams and jellies. And I haven't even mentioned the homemade wines and liqueurs. Not everybody is issued with an invitation to enter my boudoir. That honour must, definitely, be earned.

CHILDPROOF

Every child must have a clean environment . . .

Nursing mothers should eat organic food so
that the mother's milk will be a clean source
of nourishment for the suckling infant. In the past,
in Western societies, there was a kitchen custom of
a nursing or pregnant woman getting the pick of the
best food in the home, ahead of the male. This
practice led to healthier children.

The colostrum was considered to be the most vital
food on the menu for a newborn child. Colostrum
is the first flow of mother's milk produced for
nursing an infant. It is loaded with special proteins,
tailored fats, complex sugars and antibodies. This
is a *grand cru* brain and health food. It lays down the
foundation to health and increased intelligence.

Most mothers childproof the house when toddlers
are on the move. They can get anywhere and everywhere. They can do the unimaginable: they can come

to harm. A home also has to be childproofed against harmful chemicals that will change the DNA of the growing youngster, leading to disease and cancers in the future.

Fish, meats and cheese you bring home wrapped in plastic should be re-wrapped in greaseproof paper or, preferably, placed into a glass container and put into the fridge. These foods contain oleic, linoleic and linolenic fatty acids, essential nutrients that will dissolve the toxic phthalates out of plastic wrap. The phthalates then migrate into the food. When you eat them, the plastic molecules as monomers relocate themselves in the endoplasmic reticulum of your cells, where they accumulate. They wait for an opportunity to cause cancer. This may take up to twenty years. Children are the most vulnerable.

Keep the kitchen simple: wood, metal, glass and heat-cured ceramics. These products are stable. They do not break down easily.

The warm cycle of the dishwasher hydrates the air in the kitchen. This hydrated air dissolves and captures toxins from non-natural furniture and appliances, plastic polymers and fire retardants in cloth. Other polymers and their glues from plywoods and furniture will dissolve also. These toxins, even in low concentrations, affect children because they are growing so rapidly.

Children need clean water. The younger the child, the cleaner the water he or she needs. Almost 97 percent of the potable water of North America is contaminated with medicines ranging from heart medications to estrogens to antibiotics. Pesticides and veterinary medicines of industrial farming leak into the water supply. The sea is also changing from the practices of cage fish farming and the use of antibiotics in fish food. Water needs to be filtered through molecular-level-sized pores to remove these toxins. Carbon filters are excellent, too, but they need to be frequently changed.

A child's skin is sensitive and delicate. Do not wash it with soaps that are laced with antibiotics. A little dirt on the skin will do a lot less harm than a super-clean skin saturated with antibiotics. There are good bacteria living on skin. They are needed for the healthy maintenance of the skin.

One of the good-news stories in the last few years is the innovation in cleaning products made from white vinegar, baking soda and natural plant extracts.

These are non-toxic for the toddler and household pets. You can make cleaning products from these substances yourself, or read the labels on commercial efforts.

The power of the purse holds the balance for business. The more money that is spent on non-toxic household items, the cleaner our environment will be. Remember that.

BAKING SODA

The best medicine you can keep in your house . . .

It is a secret. It is silent. It sits in your kitchen cupboard between the table salt and black pepper. In Asia it divides the soya sauce and star anise from the sesame seed oil and Sichuan peppercorns.

Baking soda, or bicarbonate of soda, is the green machine of the future. Even the very preparation and manufacture of this marvellous household product has a carbon-sequestering action because it is prepared from naturally occurring sodium carbonate, also called thermonatrite, together with water and carbon dioxide.

Baking soda is well known to cooks. The famous soda bread of the Irish comes to the table as a nutty-tasting, light brown bread, which is not so easy to make. The effervescence of carbon dioxide at 200°C (400°F) in baking should lighten the dough, giving the bread the correct open texture.

Baking soda is the most important chemical buffer system in human and animal bodies. A buffer is a chemical or biochemical that, in solution, can neutralize an acid or the opposite, an alkali. It acts like a chemical mop, neutralizing the corrosive actions of either the acid or the alkali. So if a drop of acid or alkali gets on your skin or clothing you reach for the baking soda box as soon as possible to eliminate the burning effect.

Brushing your teeth with baking soda once in a while will keep them white and clean. If you have inflamed or injured gums, rinse with a quarter teaspoon of baking soda in a cup of warm water to soothe the sore gums and help them heal. The solution should be held in the mouth and flushed around the teeth, then spat out and followed by a quick rinse of warm water. I use a baking soda solution rinse once in a while as a tonic for my mouth bacteria, keeping them in balance to do their probiotic work of teeth and gum protection.

Life is such a rush nowadays that many people take antacids for stomach problems, stress and strain. Some of these tablets and powders are made of baking soda, which buffers the hydrochloric acid reflux of the stomach. When stressed, the stomach produces more acid. This is known as nervous stomach. While it is better for the body to sit back and count to ten, or to one thousand, if the case merits it, many people prefer to pop the pill or the powder.

Bicarbonate of soda in solution is used as a skin wash to very effectively get rid of candidiasis, which is a disease caused by the yeast candida. Candida yeasts form part of the normal ecology of the skin surfaces of the human body. When such yeasts get out of control, as they do very easily with modern industrial foods, stress, and overuse of antibiotics, it can become a problem. A solution of half a teaspoon of bicarbonate of soda in a cup of warm water can be used as a rinse and left to dry naturally on the skin. This acts as a shield or molecular buffer on the skin. In this way, it is an effective fungicide.

Summer in North America brings with it a quota of mosquitoes, blackflies, bees and various wasps. Many bite or sting, causing considerable discomfort. Wasp and bee stings respond to a paste of bicarbonate of soda on the skin to relieve the pain and buffer the

poisons released by the insects. A solution of half
a teaspoon of baking soda in a cup of warm water
gives relief from the bites of all the other critters.
Let the solution dry on the skin and the blighters
will leave you alone because they will not smell your
pheromones, at least not for a while.

Now we are on to something much more
embarrassing. Sometimes there are odours that
the discreet housekeeper wants to make disappear.
Place a partially opened box of baking soda in
the bathroom, or god forbid, in the bedroom and
unpleasant fragrances will be absorbed by the soda.
Place an opened box next to the kitty litter container,
too, for the relief of the household.

If teenagers or children are learning to cook,
place a large box of baking soda within reach of the
stove. There is nothing that quenches a thirsty fire
like a big box of baking soda. It is the main ingredient
in many fire extinguishers.

The gardeners of the house can also reach for the
box. In the fall when spring bulbs are being planted,
sprinkle baking soda lightly on top of your most
prized bulbs. This will de-scent them, foiling the
local squirrel population. The squirrels' noses cannot

smell the flesh of the bulb when there is baking soda on top.

While we are on the topic of the garden, summers are becoming hot, humid and muggy all over the world. Reach for the soda box when you see the plant fungus called powdery mildew in your garden. It shows up as a whitish film on the surface of soft leaves. This little plant killer has just made its way into the precious gardens of England and Ireland. Make a spray from 1 tablespoon of baking soda per litre (4 cups) of warm water. Spray the surface of the plant. Smile. It will be better now.

And for the final item, baking soda is the best and finest environmental cleaner on Earth. It will even work to clean the delicate shells of eggs. The chemist in me loves baking soda. It is my personal secret to share.

How to Boil Water

An increasingly essential skill . . .

Mother Earth, your children have forgotten how to boil water. When the new water main broke in Boston in 2010, and the order to boil water came through the media, people went into a panic. The radio stations were inundated with calls, asking the universal question "How do you boil water?"

You need to know how to boil water to make it safe to drink. And, more important, you must know the reasons why.

Water makes life go around. The water of rivers, streams and lakes is called fresh water. Deep aquifers underground hold ancient fossil water, which is really unique and pure. A salty version is in the ocean. A similar salty version is in your blood, which pumps through your heart and motors you along in your life. Water is in the makeup of every cell of your body, all of which mix and match to form the beauty

that is you. Your life, itself, depends on water.
Population pressure is increasing the demand
for water and the supply is limited. Climate change
is moving water around, dropping the levels of
rivers and lakes and increasing the mass volume
of the ocean. The continental aquifers of the world
are shrinking.

Once upon a time much of our water was clean.
I remember drinking from streams and slate-lined
wells. "Clean" for water means that it is made up of
only two things, oxygen and hydrogen. Nothing else.
Outside of a laboratory, water is no longer clean.
All the stuff that goes down the toilet, all the stuff
that gets put into the air and all the stuff that gets
cut down with the forests, ends up in water. Some
of the contamination gets cleaned out of the water
during sewage treatment. You drink the rest. It
looks clean. But it is not. It carries chlorine as an
antiseptic, for starters.

When a water main breaks in Canada due to frost,
earthquakes or other reasons, bacteria contaminate
the water. You will not be able to see them on any
given day, but if there is a lot of bacteria and debris
in the water, it becomes turbid and does not look

clean. It becomes more like a thin soup. In warmer weather this soup thickens. This is not good for you, your children, your cats, your dogs, or any other household pet you might have, even a husband.

There will be more boil water orders in North America and across the world because money is tight and the infrastructure of our towns and cities is crumbling. So when you get an official government boil water advisory, do not drink water from the tap. Do not even brush your teeth with it. Get a kettle and fill it. Then put it on the element and turn it on. Wait until the water begins to boil. Of course there is an old wives' tale that "a watched pot never boils." Not true! It does. Wait a minute or two more until the water in the kettle is at a good rolling boil. By this I mean that you can see large bubbles of air rise up and pop on the surface of the water. After three minutes of boiling, turn off the element and let the water cool down for use in drinking or cooking or brushing your teeth.

Boiling water like this causes the molecular structure of the water to rub itself together as if it were washing itself. All the filth gets dropped to the bottom of the kettle into a solid known as a precipitate. Sometimes this precipitate is white and caked, a chemical called calcium carbonate from hard water. It is fairly harmless. Sometimes the calcium is stained a brown colour, which means that there is iron in the precipitate. Throw away these droppings in the bottom of the kettle. Just drink the upper layers of water. It is cleaner.

Now for the bad news. Dirty water from a broken pipe has a good chance of having pathogenic bacteria in it. If you drink these bad boys you bring them inside your body. They prosper and replicate there. Viruses, such as the polio virus, might be in the water, too. There are many more pathogens out there to give you nightmares. Some can kill and others can maim. But boiling water destroys these pathogens.

So learn how to boil water. It is a simple way of being safe and sound. And when I visit, use it to make me a good cup of tea. Boil the kettle. Warm the teapot. Add a spoon of loose tea for the pot and a spoon for every person who is drinking the tea. And for heaven's sake, use a tea cosy. It's the least I will expect.

Bathing Beauties

Skip a shower once in a while . . .

The ancient Romans had an extraordinary love of bathing. The need for water was great. The Empire put its engineers to the task of plumbing water from the lakes, rivers and streams to build public and private baths. The fresh water came from everywhere in aqueducts whose stone arches went across farmland, towns and valleys.

The engineers put the master masons to work. Stone was hewn into ashlar that fit together so tightly even a sheet of paper could not squeeze between the seams of the finished stonework. These pools were used for bathing and relaxed gossip. When the day's work was over, the Romans plunged into their beloved watering holes in all the organic splendour of their birthday suits.

The bathwater was hot, deliciously so, with just

the right amount of heat to make the well-worked body relax. To achieve this state of affairs, the Romans built a network of clay pipes around the bath. These held water, too, which was heated separately by a fire some distance away. The clay pipes were sealed with naturally occurring clay called bentonite that expanded with water to become watertight, enclosing the entire unit. The clay pipes and the bentonite held the heat for a very long time so that bathers could enjoy the cool of the evening in warm water with very little work or worry.

The baths of the privileged received extra care. Archaeologists are still digging up beautiful tiles with glorious designs and a rainbow of colours. The skilled artists who produced these ceramics knew what they were doing for a clientele who could appreciate and promote their works of art.

Then the roses were used. To celebrate an occasion, the very rich brought in a shipment of rose petals to be used as confetti. *Rosa damascena,* or the damask rose, was an outstandingly fragrant and popular red rose that was grown by horti-culturalists outside of Rome as a mass-market item. After the rose petals were sprinkled liberally, togas were taken off so that the fat and the very slim could together slip into the warm waters.

North America, Europe and many parts of Asia are like Rome. The very rich have rain rooms where the shower points are plumbed into the ceiling, the walls and sometimes into the floor. The temperature of the water can be adjusted by a click of a switch to run the range of hot to cold. There are designer washing rooms out there with mosaic seats of incredible art. Even the less fortunate indulge in every form of bathing with jet foam corner baths and outdoor hot tubs.

The rich and the poor of the world are washing away their health. It is going down the drain. This is literally true. The human skin is a watertight envelope, protected by a series of glands called the sebaceous glands that feed the skin a form of fat called sebum to keep it smooth and supple. Dissolved in this sebum is another fat vital for the health of the body. The floating fat is a watchdog. It is vitamin D, the deoxy form known as the sunshine vitamin. This vitamin is also called a precursor vitamin because it waits on the exposed surface of the skin for the sun to shine. Then vitamin D goes into action and changes

itself chemically and structurally. A long shot of
sunshine or a small flash of ultraviolet light will
break the double bonds of carbon down to a single
bond. This little change is all that is needed to
produce the full-blooded vitamin D that every single
human being on the planet relies upon for health.

Vitamin D is not just one vitamin, but part of
a family of closely related members. There are
vitamins D, D_1, D_2, D_3 and D_4. These all have a
wonderful structure called bipolar. Both ends
can receive sunshine and transform it into energy.
This energy, in turn, forms a molecule that has
a different action in the body. Science is trying to
more fully understand the function of vitamin D.

The vitamin, after being acted upon by sunshine,
dives into the human body to work as a hormone
and a fence against disease. Vitamin D also mediates
in calcium absorption in the gut. Without the
vitamin, calcium will not be absorbed into the body.
Once it is in the body, vitamin D is directly involved
in bone building and in maintaining the entire
skeleton. Every single muscle cell must have calcium,
too, for action and reaction. Without vitamin D
a disease called rickets shows itself with weak and

bending bones, especially of the legs because they carry the weight of the body. Good sleep and diabetes are also managed by calcium and therefore vitamin D.

Vitamin D as a family goes on to regulate the metabolism of calcium throughout the human body, fine-tuning it for an active life. It is also a precursor hormone, which means that it is a building block for the making of other human hormones.

We have become much too clean. We have washed the best of our health down the drain.

Antibiotics

Respect them for the killers they are . . .

Just examine the word "antibiotic." *Anti*, of course, means against, and *bioté* is Greek for life, so the word itself means anti-life. Antibiotics are killing machines in the ever-so-small world of molecules. There are antibiotics that are part of nature, found in the land, sea and air. These are chemicals with an edge. And there are synthetic antibiotics with a true killer's instinct that are being used and abused on a daily basis.

Day-old chicks have enough food in their system to keep them going for a day. They are then fed starter feed, which is finely milled bits of grain. Starter feed is laced with antibiotics and is fed to chicks for six to eight weeks. This medicated feed continues for the life of a battery hen, raised for the single purpose of egg production.

Cows, pigs and horses are fed antibiotics, too. Their urine, bearing this medication, passes into the groundwater system. Cows are milked. Sometimes if the milking is delayed, the lactating cow can get mastitis, requiring prescriptive antibiotics on top of the medication in their feed. Pigs, too, receive antibiotics to suppress their intestinal flora so that weight gain is greater. Cattle, also. Sheep receive fewer antibiotics because they are hardier and generally not raised in confined spaces.

In the oceans or estuaries, fish farms use antibiotics in their feed. The fish farms grow caged fish and shellfish. Only a few decades ago the fish and shellfish we ate were caught in the wild. Their health was protected by nature. Now medicated feed is on the menu so that the caged fish will not get sick and cause an epidemic outside in the wild stock that live in the same water only a few feet away.

Cheeses are caught in the same trap; antibiotics are added to the process to create a long shelf life, all for the bottom line. This is just for starters.

I am reminded of a message that went across the medical world thirty-five years ago requesting physicians to halt the excessive prescribing of antibiotics. I remember reading the piece in a state of exhaustion after a bout of surgery. My greens had been flung into a common basket. I had my street clothes on, my mind for some reason still in the sterile mode of the operating room and all of its problems. The worry about antibiotics got caught in the gill net of my consciousness and stayed there.

A day or so later, I bumped into a girlfriend in town. She had an important job and should have been working. I asked her why the holiday. She told me that her children were both sick with a cold and she had taken them to the doctor for antibiotics. I suggested that bed rest and liquids might be a better regimen. She just laughed. I couldn't figure out how to tell her that the overuse of antibiotics casts a long shadow.

At the same time my nearest neighbour retired from flying. He decided to become a dairy farmer and bought a milk quota. He set about protecting his investment with antibiotics. He bought them by the caseload to dose his forty or so black-and-white Friesian cows. By giving them antibiotics he hoped that he would bypass the problems of mastitis and bump up his milk production to receive a bigger cheque. In the meantime the antibiotics passed from his cows into their milk and then on into the creams, butter, yogurts, whey butter, sour cream, curds, cheeses, skimmed and whole milk and ice cream products made from that milk.

What kind of point am I trying to make? I am trying to say that like all killers, antibiotics should be respected. They should not be used willy-nilly. They absolutely should not be added to liquid soaps for use on the delicate skin of the body. Nor should they be added into animal food nor used as a wash to clean the surfaces of furniture and food. They should not be sprayed in orchards. They should not be dispersed in the ocean and they should be removed from drinking water with fine carbon filtration. Antibiotics should be treated as target medicines to treat specific bacterial infection, by trained professionals who know why, and more important, what they are doing.

I am saying all of this because of the dreaded term "superbugs." The dark shadow of overuse brings antibiotic resistance into our daily vocabulary, and that resistance lays the foundations for epidemics and global pandemics. No detective of science can forecast when the wrong prion or the right bacteria will make its deadly move. One thing we can all do is not abuse antibiotics, because we will never know when we will really need them. Then it might well be a matter of life or death, for a great number of people.

SORE EYES

Carrots and computers go together...

When I was a little girl of six or seven, I loved to go for walks with my mother. We would strike out to a destination hand in hand. Very often the choice of location was mine.

Like most children, I had a favourite place of such glamour and beauty that it held me enthralled for days after each visit. It was a long avenue of golden chain trees, known in Canada more often as laburnum, set into a stone-terraced garden. The long locks of sweet-smelling, pea-like flowers dangled above your head while the pavement was a bright yellow carpet of spent blooms. I felt they were enchanted.

One afternoon in June a terrible accident happened. I shudder even now, when I think of it. A car passed by. The driver flicked a cigarette butt out the window. I was looking at the laburnums as the cigarette travelled through the air. The burning tip flared, bounced against a stone of the terrace and snapped into my eye. First, I did not know what was producing the terrible pain in my eye. I do not remember what happened after that except that I had a year's worth of visits to the eye doctor because of the damage done to my eye.

The eyes work as photo receptors; that is, they take in reflected light and focus it to produce a visual image. This image is subsequently stored in the brain for recall and use as needed.

Suburban living with artificial lighting and fluorescent computer screens demand a high standard of sight from the working eye. To keep pace, the eye must be well fed with foods from a healthy diet that contain vitamin A. This vitamin is essential for healthy sight because it is the building block for the working machinery of sight itself. However, because the storage facilities in the liver are somewhat limited, it can also become a toxin to the body.

The gracious carrot comes to the rescue. Carrots contain carotene, which is the yellow-to-orange colouring of this root vegetable. Carotene is known as a vitamin A precursor. This means that a carrot, cooked or raw, is eaten and digested. In the gut there is a covey of bacteria, like maids-in-waiting. They inspect the carotene molecule and check supplies with the liver and blood. If vitamin A is needed, they snip the carotene into two identical pieces with an enzyme, delivering two molecules of vitamin A as the result. Vitamin A then may be shelved for storage in the liver or put into the mass transit of the blood, bound to a piece of protein called RBP or retinol-binding protein, and sent on its way to bolster the eyes for seeing.

Carotene or vitamin A precursor is found in many other plant foods also, especially the green leaves of fresh spinach, Swiss chard and beet greens. Usually carotene occurs with chlorophyll or the green matter of plants. There is a nice little trick that can cheaply increase the carotene content of all winter storage squash, which is another source. Bathe the squash in light at a 10°C (50°F) temperature for three weeks. This matures the skin of the squash and increases the carotene content of its flesh considerably. The squash is then placed in dark winter storage for later use. All fruits and most vegetables contain some carotene.

Other full-blooded sources of the fat-soluble vitamin A are liver, milk, butter, cheese, eggs and fish, especially fish liver oils. These sources do not need the attention of attendant bacteria in the gut, but can travel on their own way into storage and wait until they receive their call to be used by the body.

The eyes also need another helping hand when they have to adapt from light to darkness or from darkness to light. Some people have trouble with this change of circumstance, and the adaptive ability of the eyes is not all it should be, especially during the winter months when the eyes become conditioned to low light levels that can change in a second when flashed by the strong headlights of an oncoming car, or if the eyes are tired or strained from overuse by working at computer screens all day.

The eyes also take longer to get accustomed to changing light conditions as they age. This adaptation might take up to a minute or two even in a familiar bedroom or kitchen. The blueberry, *Vaccinium angustifolium,* or the Saskatoon berry, *Amelanchier alnifolia*, both carry quercetin, a compound that acts as a fine capillary protector. These fruits help the eye to see. The unusual sugar content of these berries feeds an energy cycle in the eye to make the eye more effective.

Caring for your sight is simple; just eat a good serving of carrots followed by fresh blueberries as dessert. You might even enjoy it as much as I do.

Avoidance Therapy

Learn to read the labels of the food you eat . . .

Some conventionally grown fruits and vegetables are always more toxic to eat than others. They are more toxic because of the regime of fungicides, herbicides and pesticides used in their propagation and growth. After harvest, some are sprayed or gassed or misted with plant hormones like ethylene during transportation from one country to another, to either stall or control the ripening process and to control insects and fungal growth to ensure good looks for instant sale at their destination. Others get a coat of paraffin, a waxing that would make the dining table shine.

Areas of the world that receive more rain during the growing season are forced to apply more spray and more often, for it to be effective. The wetter the area, the more toxic the food it produces. There are also countries whose regulations governing

pesticide sale, application and handling differ
from the country of retail. Some pesticides are
systemic, which means they become trapped within
the flesh when sprayed on the surface. These sprays
cannot be washed off with water; even soap or alcohol
will not do the trick. They have changed the chemical
imprint of the food and when you eat it, that change
goes right into the body, which has to cope with this
new molecular toxin. Sometimes it can but other
times it cannot, because all people are not equal,
biochemically. Occasionally the toxin can lay
dormant in the fat tissue of the body, slowly
accumulating with time.

The most contaminated foods in supermarkets
are non-organic potatoes, especially winter storage
varieties, followed closely by apples, pears and
plums. Sweet cherries, raspberries, blackberries,
peaches and nectarines come next. Depending on
the year, strawberries and blackberries are close
on their tracks. In a hot, dry year there is less need
for fungicides. Sour cherries, cranberries and
blueberries require less spray than other fruits.
In fact, the large growers here in Canada are
conducting their own research and development

toward full organic production of these small fruits. Foreign grapes are often sprayed with fungicide in transit to reduce mould. The buyer can detect such sprays as long white streaks on the fruit, as opposed to the talc of wild yeast.

Spring vegetables that grow rapidly to maturity in the cool, short days of the season are less toxic. These are asparagus, both green and blanched, summer turnips and their greens and all varieties of kohlrabies and radishes. Vegetables like carrots, parsnips, rutabagas, burdock, scorzonera and salsify, including the winter storage radishes, require little spray. Beets, both early and winter storage kinds, of all colours, and Swiss chard are grown with very little pesticide application.

Snow, sugar snap and other peas are usually organic if their seeds have not been drenched in fungicides. The same goes for bush beans, pole beans and any other climbing bean, especially those whose beans are shelled for dry beans. Fresh beans hold an off-flavour if they have been sprayed, and they rot rapidly. Lettuce salad mixes, micro greens and spinach are usually organic, due to the cold hardiness of the mixture. They can dodge insect infestation and fungal diseases.

The summer greens, collards, rapini, Brussels sprouts, Asian greens, broccoli, cauliflower and cabbages, both red and white, are easy to grow without sprays. Generally the more northern the source, the cleaner they are. They can also be mechanically protected by row covers to keep cabbage butterflies away. In addition, cabbages grow from the inside out, so the outer leaves can be discarded, leaving the cleaner centres; the natural wax or cuticle of the leaf will help shed the spray.

The mid-summer vegetables require less spray. Their main requirement for health is sufficient heat units from the sun to ripen them. Occasionally a number of fungal diseases threaten these crops, due to weather, which cannot be controlled. All tomatoes, especially the disease-resistant types, peppers, zucchini and summer squash, eggplants, cucumbers, winter squash and pumpkins, receive fewer pesticides for the simple reason that many of the common sprays damage their crisp appearance for market and sale. Most of the heritage tomatoes that are now available in season are raised organically because they need pampering to retain flavour.

Local garlic is usually grown organically, and has a superior flavour and keeping quality. Leeks, too, are mostly organic. But onions are a different matter since they are already one of the species affected by climate change and overheated soils, which has given rise to a battery of new and old diseases. Pickling onions are no longer available due to disease. For the present, onions, grown in winter in southern latitudes, are less toxic than local varieties grown in Canada.

Oranges, limes, lemons, tangerines, mandarins, grapefruit, watermelon, cantaloupes, pineapples and papaya need only to be washed and dried. Bananas just require peeling. This popular fruit is under threat from disease because in the tropics the night temperatures have increased. Banana trees use the cooling air of night to recover from the searing temperatures of the day.

An increase of summer temperatures benefits the growing of sweet potatoes and yams, peppers, okra and the delicious pawpaw. The diseases for these species do not abound yet and so they can be expected to be fully organic when bought, as can the table grape and my all-time favourite fruit, the lychee nut.

Remember, if more people request and buy clean food, the prices will go down. These consumer actions will also encourage further innovation to reduce spraying and chemical contamination in our food supply for everyone.

Bee Balm

An ancient American herb becomes modern again . . .

A number of years ago the Mohawk council of
Akwesasne near Cornwall, Ontario, asked me
to assist a medicine woman, Ceci Mitchell. Ceci was
becoming famous outside of North America for
prescribing her own native pharmacopeia of traditional medicines for her peoples. Herbalists and
medical biochemists from Germany and Russia
were interested in the uses of these plants, especially
the rare ones, to apply in their own countries. Ceci
wanted all of these species named in Latin, because
it is the universal language amongst botanists.

We hiked into the areas she used for collecting.
Some of the plants we encountered I had not seen
in flower before. These were true species of the wild
growing in their own special luxury. As we walked
I noticed that the landscape of her mind remembered
past and present medicinal plants growing in certain

places. Sometimes she looked and the plants were, indeed, there. Other times she would say, while staring ahead into the distance, that the orchids would return again in seven years. She showed me her secret stash of goldenseal, *Hydrastis canadensis*, her wonder drug, and worried about its survival into the future because of weather changes.

I had seen this kind of memory before when I was a child in Ireland, in the old people who carried the knowledge of the Celtic cures. The landscape to them was different. It was as if they saw the hand of nature everywhere and remembered the special events of a holly tree, *Ilex aquifolium*, carrying a heavy load of berries in a certain year or the strawberry tree of the Druids, *Arbutus unedo*, bearing fruit or the little ladies bedstraw, *Galium verum*, ready to use in making cheese.

The medicine women of the farming communities of Ireland kept their more useful traditional medicinal plants close at hand, sometimes a few feet from the doorstep. That practice is largely gone now, but I think we should bring it back. There is one plant of the North American and Mexican virgin forests that should be kept in every household garden. It belongs to a famous family, the *Labiatae*. This family of flowering, aromatic, medicinal herbs has a history dating back before written records in Europe and central Asia.

The plant is called bee balm or wild bergamot, *Monarda didyma*. Pale blue bee balm still stalks a few of the remaining virgin forests of North America and was a favourite of the aboriginal peoples. They used the sweet green leaves containing linalool in a tea or tisane. This tea was responsible for the Boston Tea Party in 1773, a protest against the new taxes imposed by the British Empire on the black-tea-drinking habits of the colonies. The tea chests from Asia were dumped into Boston Harbor in favour of the American-grown Oswego tea. This tea, in a new dress, flavoured with bee balm, is called Earl Grey and still remains a favourite to those who shiver at the very niggle of the word "taxes."

Bee balm has a strange form of flower, shaped like a mop made up of many individual flowers. The original colour is sky blue or white, but a wide range going from blood red to deep purple and various shades of mauve are readily available. Inside each individual little floret is a fresh, flowing nectary that oozes sugary sap. Hummingbirds and bees simply love this sap, so if you grow bee balm you can expect a lot of these visitors.

All gardeners should care for a plant of bee balm. Its fragrance is released by the slightest touch. The glandular hairs on the soft leaves release a form of aerosol medicine that opens up the lungs for deeper breathing. This airborne medicine wafts around the outside of the home, drifts in through open windows and benefits everybody inside.

Since ancient times, Europe, Asia and in particular the Arab cultures of the world used a relative of bee balm called lemon balm, *Melissa officinalis*. It is a seriously strong medicinal herb used for the relief of anxiety and depression and is still used as a sedative tea. It was once placed into bathing waters to treat restlessness and that almost universal event of modern living, nervous tachycardia. Nowadays, lemon balm has made its way into proprietary cordials and liqueurs. In Europe it is also known as thé de France.

Household gardens can be small green paradises, resting places for the entire family to sit, relax and recover from the tensions of living. There has never been a greater need for humans to keep a few treasured plants near their doorsteps. Brushing by a patch of bee balm will liberate a free plume of aerosol medicine that will make you feel good and perhaps more human again.

There is just one more thing. Bee balm can also be dried in the sun and used in an herbal pillow for sweeter sleep and deeper dreams. Try it!

Cheap Chick

Help the hummingbirds to survive across the world . . .

S ome people call them by a pet name: hummers.
I love that name. They are one of my favourite
birds in the garden. As soon as the frost of winter
goes, I am on the lookout for them. A strange thing
happens to me every spring. The name hummingbird
comes very strongly into my mind as if they are
sending up a non-verbal message from the Deep
South. I immediately wash out the feeding stations
I've kept in storage in the pumphouse, fill them,
hang them and wait. The hummingbirds arrive
within twenty-four hours.

I maintain four separate hummingbird stations
in the garden. They are always in the same place,
distanced from one another because hummingbirds
are territorial. One goes on the front of the house.
To the left of this feeding station, just a half metre
(18 inches) away, I grow a single cordon apple tree,

pruned to the height of the lower roof of the house. This tree is a landing site for the birds to rest and to groom before they feed. It also catches and reflects all the heat of the house. It is a warm spot to refresh returning birds. They always come to this place. I can see them from the kitchen.

I place the second feeder on a low branch of a white ash, *Fraxinus americana*. This branch grows above my black peony border, *Paeonia lactiflora* 'Chocolate Soldier,' which I have cross-bred for their chocolate smell. From the position of the ash tree, the hummingbirds can service the black walnut *allée*. These are nut trees Christian and I have developed for flavour over the years. They produce nectars and honeydews that feed the hummingbirds. The birds also hang nests in the lower limbs of these trees.

The third and fourth feeders are placed in the Medicine Walk on the pergola. These areas are open to the vegetable garden nearby. My gladioli collection is always part of the vegetable garden. It consists of very early flowers, mid-season flowers and late, hardy flowers that I have bred. The hummingbirds have a feast with these flowers. Then there is the bean castle that Christian and I manage to erect each spring, a pyramid that rises to around 3 or 4 metres (or 12 feet). It is made of cedar poles and baling twine, planted with unusual scarlet runner beans such as the variety 'Painted Lady.' Inside this bean castle there is an observation seat for children to eat ice cream and watch hummers in secret.

Hummingbirds are one of the marvels of our natural world. They push the limits of flight to the edge of scientific possibility with their size and their energy requirements to produce their speed. They can hover in the same spot for a very long time and they can do something that no other bird can do: fly backwards.

Typically hummingbirds overwinter in a warm place like Mexico or Panama. They return north following the movement of spring and its flowers up the face of the North American continent to court with their pendulum dance, to breed and rear their young. In Eurasia, they do the same thing. Recently in England, gardeners have been reporting a change in the behaviour of these birds. They are appearing in places they have never been seen before. Their arrivals are earlier, also.

Because hummingbirds are such high-energy

creatures they must take their food in its most basic form, sugar. They evolved millennia ago to visit the sugar factories of the plant world. These are called nectaries and arise at the base of each petal or around the perimeter of the female portion of the flower. Nectaries are glands that produce sugars with high mineral content. These sugars change the physics of flow and can bead to a greater height than water. The hummingbird takes advantage of this by dipping its beak and feeding.

There are other sources of food with which the hummingbird is familiar. These are extra floral nectaries, glands on other parts of the plant that produce a high-value product filled with sugar. In recent years, biologists caught another first for the record. They filmed hummingbirds catching and eating mosquitoes. So it seems they do enjoy a little protein with their sugared drink.

Hummingbirds will readily come to feeders. The feeders should be made of glass and not plastic. The feeding area must have a little stand for them to settle to drink, and the artificial feeding flower should be red with scarlet petals. The feeder should be placed out of the reach of Bristles the cat. And the piece of nylon string or wire used to hang the feeder from a hook should have a daub of petroleum jelly or Tree Tanglefoot paste on it to keep the ants away from the sugar solution and from going inside.

Hummingbird food for home feeders is very cheap to make. All you need is white table sugar and a transparent 1-litre (2-cup) glass measuring cup. Put a cup of white sugar into the measuring cup and add warm water slowly until the sugar is almost dissolved. Stir the sugar mixture until it loses the look of pure water and has a swirly appearance to it. Let the solution rest in the measuring cup for five minutes or so while you are doing something else.

When you come back, the solution should have a few crystals of sugar lying at the bottom of the cup. If they are not there, slowly add a bit more sugar until they are. On the other hand, if there is too much sugar lying at the bottom of the cup, simply add a bit more warm water, slowly stirring so that the sugar at the bottom almost dissolves. You'll know it's right when a few crystals are left behind on the bottom of the cup.

This is called making a saturated solution. Such solutions are commonly made in a chemical laboratory using ingredients other than sugar, but the idea is the same. Saturation is a balanced harmony between the sugar and the water. It is the same harmony that exists in plant nectar. It will keep and not go off, much like honey or jam. Now you are ready to pour the solution into the clean hummingbird feeder. If there is any sugar solution left over, store it in the fridge in a clean glass container. Use it to top up the feeder until you need to make another batch.

Hummingbirds cannot feed from double flowers because the extra set of petals acts as a barrier to their ability to penetrate the flower and fly or hover at the same time. They love open flowers of the old-fashioned kind like single hollyhocks, hibiscus, runner beans, gladioli, trumpet creepers, bee balm, all of the petunias, impatiens, all of the globe thistles, and sea holly. The lilies are also a favourite. They love your flowers and will visit your feeder, too. They will thank you for your act of mercy with a hum from their incredible wings and a flash of fire from their gentle breast.

Hair Care

A gift for the birds . . .

Over half of the world has gone urban, according to the Global Health Observatory of the World Health Organization. People have migrated from the carbon castle of nature, turned their backs on the feeding fields and set their sights on a concrete kingdom, their new home. Money dangles like a golden carrot in front of the donkey, always too far away for most to grasp.

Every house in every city can still do something for the natural world around them. Every city garden and every balcony can make an offering to the great migration of birds and butterflies that pass silently overhead from spring to fall, and back again.

To reproduce, a bird must build a nest. A nest can take many forms, from the egg cup of the hummingbird to the stick platform of the osprey, to the few mottled brown leaves of the whippoorwill on the open ground. Even the ordinary laying hen that produces brown and white eggs for the kitchen table will surprise you if left to her own devices. She will carve a small oval cave in the side of a hill and lay her clutch of eggs on the earth. She then sits on the eggs, carefully spreading out her feathered body to trap the heat she produces to keep her eggs at the perfect temperature for incubation. She is absolutely faithful to this task and if the heat reflection from the soil makes one or two of her eggs a little over temperature she will use her beak to gently nudge the egg to roll exactly 180 degrees to cool its over-warm face to guard the embryo inside. Her baby chicks emerge in twenty-one days and then she must mother them all.

For wild birds in an urban setting, incubation becomes a problem. This is also true for regions of the countryside where industrial farming takes place. In the past, birds pinched hair from the wild animals they found sleeping as they searched for nesting materials. Muskox and buffalo had the best quality of fibre, but nowadays birds will steal back hairs from a dog sleeping in the sun. The dogs never even feel the nip.

The bird carefully weaves the hairs into a nest
with twigs, grasses, mosses and lichens to make
a cup. Some, like the vireo, do a colour blending
of the material for absolute privacy and secrecy.
The cups that hold the newly laid eggs are themselves
important. The structure must hold warmth and
maintain its temperature to the degree required
by the nesting bird. Hair is an excellent natural
insulator. The fibres can both attract or deflect the
heat of the sun and help control nesting temperatures
for successful egg incubation.

Apart from the hummingbirds and orioles who are
master weavers, suspending a pendant nest from the
branch tips of the America elm, there are important
songbirds that have a need for hair. The chipping
sparrow is an example. This bird arrives early into
the garden with its beautiful white eyebrows and
musical trill. Once the chicks have been raised to
young adults, the chipping sparrow pays for its board
by eating an insect menu that cleans your garden free
of pests for the following year. Once upon a time in
Canada, they were called hair birds because they
mastered the use of horsehair pulled from the tails
and manes of workhorses. Now, with these beasts of

burden in decline, the birds look to sleeping animals, but human hair will do the trick.

Next spring go out and buy a coconut. Drill a hole in it and drain off the coconut milk. This milk can go into the fridge and become an ingredient for vegan ginger squash soup, with its lingering aftertaste of coconut. Cut the coconut in half. Remove the meat and snack on it with nuts and raisins. Return to the piece with the drilled hole and make it bigger, about 5 centimetres (2 inches) in diameter. Then wire the two pieces back together so that the coconut looks whole again. Collect the cat's combing or the dog's brushing and stuff it into the coconut. Your own hair, long or short, blonde or black, will do, too. Roll the hair into a ball before stuffing it into the shell. Then place the coconut at the base of a shrub or hang it from a tree or a wire. If you have a balcony, put it on top of the soil of one of your flower containers. You can even set it somewhere in your local park.

Then, wait for your reward. One spring morning when you least expect it you will see a songbird with a white eyebrow. The little chipping sparrow is back from the heat of Nicaragua or the Baja peninsula of California. He will fly to an elevation of a tree branch or to a building to perform his song. The music will stop your breath. In that moment of beauty you will travel to eternity with the notes of the trill. Your whole day will be uplifted with that simple song of the chipping sparrow.

Cat's Thyme

Cats need their own special food from nature . . .

S ometimes I feel much closer to my animals than
to any human being. A pet can read your soul
with such clarity that it is comforting. The piercing
loneliness of mental solitude vanishes with one
purr or a cat's chin leaning on your arm.

I have had two cats in my life that were
extraordinary, both second-hand as strays. They
settled down quite comfortably together in front
of my Findlay Oval stove. Somehow, a roving Tom
left his calling card with my two ladies, who
produced a litter apiece in the due course of
time. A box at the bottom of my closet was the
chosen nest. Spookie gave birth easily but La Bandita,
who was younger, had problems. I came home
to find Spookie pushing hard with both paws on
La Bandita's belly with each contraction until every
one of her kittens came.

If that was not enough! The two females took turns mousing out in the garden. While one cat took over nursing the commonage of kittens, the other hunted, one on and one off duty until the kittens were reared. Their behaviour gave me a new respect for my pets and for anybody else's pet, in fact.

In my house, cats and dogs live a much longer life than is normal. They are healthy, too. Spookie reached twenty-three years. My vet always comments on this when he does his annual injection regime. There are reasons why this is true. The reasons are outside growing in the garden, sweet herbs especially planted for them. And what's more, my pets know it.

The first plant grows wild. It is from Eurasia, but it established itself all over the northern hemisphere long ago. I carefully leave a few young plants for the cats every spring. They can roll on them, eat them and crush them into a mush for all I care, for they are entirely the cats' business. For the winter months I bundle some dried bunches of the plant into an old sock. Catnip is the common name, the Latin *Nepeta cataria*. It produces thymol and a mixture of oils, the principal constituent of which is called nepetalactone. I suspect they stimulate the pleasure centres in the cat's brain by activating endorphins. In any case, they enable complete relaxation in the cat, which is a form of muscle resting state that is extremely beneficial to all felines.

The other plant I propagate, especially for dogs and cats, is a ground cover that functions like an outdoor carpet. They can walk on it. They can roll in it or scratch it and the plant will not care because the leaves themselves are numerous and very tiny, attached to wire-like stems that creep along the ground and over rocks. For that reason they are perfect to plant close to patio flags and walkways. The smokey blue-grey leaves and profusion of tiny pink flowers are beautiful. As the day length shortens, the foliage changes to a rich rose colour that lasts until the following spring. I'm describing a special species of thyme whose origins are unknown but botanists suspect that it is a perennial herb of somewhere in Europe or Asia. The Latin name for this fragrant herb is *Thymus pseudolanuginosus*.

This remarkable herb produces thymol from an essential oil that occurs in the tiny leaves. This thymol mixture has strong antiseptic properties for the fur of the cat or dog, as well as antibiotic and fungicidal properties, priming the fur for health. In addition, the animal eats the herb as an anthelminthic to clear any parasites or worms out of the intestinal tract.

The act of walking on a thyme carpet releases the thymol from the oil glands in the leaves and liberates it as a vapour into the air. This moves up the dogs' or cats' airways into the lungs, where it acts as a bronchodilator, releasing a larger amount of oxygen into circulation. This increases the cardiovascular function and also enables the lower section of the lungs to function better. Both asthma and breathing for dogs and cats are improved, relieving the effects of air pollution from which they also suffer. This is a free medicine that greatly benefits the pets and purse strings of a household.

Once upon a time all domesticated animals were part of the great wilderness of nature. They used their instincts to help preserve their lives and enable them to reproduce successfully. There are medicines in the wild that still do this for all animals. By being domesticated, dogs and cats are put into an artificial situation where their natural and native medicines are no longer available to them when they need them.

Help your pets by doing this kind of planting. It takes very little time to introduce catnip and thyme into even the smallest garden, or even to a pot on a windowsill. The benefits to the animals' health are great. And your vet bills go down! Maybe, someday in the future, urban planners will be inspired to be a little more creative and considerate of the four-legged members of their towns and cities. Perhaps they will design areas of public places filled with delights for the wet whiskers who will really appreciate them.

Dog's Life

Dogs successfully self-medicate with grass . . .

When I was a child, no other child would play with me. During the summer months in the countryside, the other kids were bigger and stronger. They ran away from me because I had a city accent. The reverse was true in the city during the school year; I had picked up the country tone. I was left alone to discover the world. I did.

I noticed that sheep ate many kinds of herbs in the meadows. I experimented with the ones they ate. Some carried the taste of peppermint; others had flavours I could not identify. The cows mowed the fields of grass and headed for the sweet clovers that emerged as a bounty from their own cow patties where these had dried and crumbled back to earth. The horses and donkeys put much more of everything into their mouths. Even the trees were not safe from their teeth, especially the green prickles of gorse.

The pigs ate the field itself, uprooting the sods
and throwing them in the air with glee before they
ingested them. Roots, soil and grass, all digested
with a burp.

So it didn't surprise me to discover that dogs, too,
have an appetite for grass. The dog is only one leap
away from the wolf in genetic terms and wolves are
so smart about so many things, one of which is
keeping the tribe together and healthy.

Dogs, big and small, have an innate knowledge
of the medicines that will keep them in shape. One
particular medicine is out there in the grass world.
The botany of grass shows that it is ancient and is in
the family *Gramineae*, of the monocotyledonous
herbaceous plants.

The Latin name of this particular grass is *Agropyron
repens*. The common name is couch grass. It is also
called quack grass, twitch grass, witch grass and
wheatgrass. In the past it was once called dog grass.
Pliny of Rome promoted it as an important medicine.
The aboriginal peoples of North America, too,
noticed that the working dogs they owned time
and time again ate a certain kind of grass to
self-medicate.

Originally from Europe and Asia, couch grass is found all over the world. In North America it grows from Alaska to Newfoundland and south into Mexico. Couch grass is disease free. The plant forms a mat, then puts out runners that can reach up to 2 metres (6 feet) in length. The white tips of the runners carry a series of digestive enzymes. They can grow through tree roots and the bulbs and corms of other plants, leaving a large round hole.

Couch grass carries a natural antibiotic for dogs. This antibiotic is a volatile oil and is contained in the leaf blade. There are salts of potassium, two sugars, triticin and inositol, together with mucilage, all of which are beneficial.

All dogs, like wolves, need to mark their territory. Smell is their trump card. It is important for them to know their boundaries and to keep an eye on all the problems that come into their four-legged world. They do this through a keen sense of smell and through the production of a strong scent in their urine. So the male dog lifts his leg to pee and the female squats to do the same thing. Pee for a dog is a universal barcode based on chemistry. Each dog produces its own fingerprint of biochemicals in its pee. Another dog can tag this ID. Such scent marking is a global monitoring system in the canine world. The dog had this system up and running well before the human loincloth became fashionable.

Pet dogs in cities, towns and in the countryside will obediently go for a walk on a leash. They will quite happily trot by your side until they come to couch grass. They will stop at a dead halt if they feel they need some. They will strain on their leash to grab an inch or two of green leaf. They will continue to snip off the pieces of grass until they feel they have had a sufficient amount. They will wait to swallow it and, if time permits, check on the local news with a good, deep sniff. Then they wag their tails and are on their way with or without you.

Couch grass is a urinary tract antiseptic. It contains potassium salts that keep the kidneys in good shape. Therefore, it prevents cystitis, the scourge of the canine world. The mucilage has a positive effect on the dog's gut along with the sugar, inositol. Both have a protective action on the pancreas, keeping it healthy. The antibiotic keeps the pee power of the dog in its natural state of excess for newsmongering.

Now, if only dogs could talk . . .

DEM BONES

Bones are the greatest organic fertilizer in the world . . .

In the woodshed, in an ink-black corner, lies a
white grain sack of abnormal size. This object
is in direct contrast to the cords of firewood that
balance with a will of their own. The top of the sack
is secured by a bow, made by me with a piece of baling
twine. Inside the sack I keep cow bones, all of them
the rounded 7-centimetre (2- to 3-inch) pieces
a butcher will have on offer. Mine were bought and
paid for, then they repaid me with beef stock before
I dried and stored them. Their final resting place
will be under my trees.

I realize that room for such a treasury of mortality
is not usually found in suburban houses. Nor do
I brag about the crypt in my woodshed. As I add to
the sack I plan their burial plots. Some go to the
fruit trees in the orchard, others to my endangered
trees to give them a boost and more again to the nut

trees who need them for longevity and nut production. They also rest .5 metres (1.5 feet) under my Fredonia black grapevines.

In North America the aboriginal peoples would plant a whole fish or fishbones under their triad of vegetables: corn, beans and squash. In Europe the tradition was to add cereal, such as oatmeal, into the planting hole as a slow-release fertilizer. In China— and most probably in many other countries as well— gardeners used night soil. Now the subject is a little too delicate. The rose gardens of the English country houses were certainly maintained by manure from the horse stables. In any case such rituals are only part of what is called in science the great nitrogen cycle.

In my garden I practice frugality, which is the natural partner of sustainability. I buy only organic bones from the butcher to make soup stock in the winter months. A selection of veggies from the root cellar gets put into that soup depending on the recipe, and as I mentioned in "Bee's Knees," the bones are washed, dried and saved.

I'm always a little anxious about the sack when the horticultural tours come to visit my garden and a stray gardener gets lost in that dark corner of my shed and comes across a bag of bones. So far, nobody thinks that I am saving up my ancestors. So far. Bones are a twenty- to twenty-five-year fertilizer. They are free. Bone meal from crushed, steamed and pulverized bones is sold commercially and is expensive and, because of its granular form, only a five- to six-year fertilizer.

When in close contact with the soil, bones are broken down by the living earth. This process is so beautifully slow that it proceeds at an excellent rate for trees and large shrubs that will live for a long time. The macro elements of potassium, nitrogen and phosphorus in bone are matched in a perfect pairing with the microelements like calcium, selenium, gold and cobalt. These are slowly transformed to soluble salts by soil bacteria, forming a leachate that pools around the growing zones of the roots. Trees have sensing mechanisms for the presence of food, and their roots will grow toward it. This is known as trophism. It is an act much like a hungry hand reaching out for a piece of food. The trees benefit immensely from these bones in my shallow soil.

When planting a nut tree like a kingnut hickory, *Carya laciniosa*, which will grow to 60 metres (200 feet), dig the hole about 45 centimetres (18 inches) deeper than normal, place six or so bones into the base of the hole and spread them away from one another. Tamp them down to stabilize them in the earth. Then place a layer of compost-enriched soil over the bones and press that down lightly. The tree is ready to plant in its resting place. Add soil and firm it down with several good waterings. Mould a lip from sod or earth about 60 centimetres (2 feet) in diameter around the tree to catch the rainfall of the growing season in a natural saucer. As the tree continues to grow, the root mass will level out the saucer area.

Each growing season, the tree will absorb nitrogen out of the bones to build protein structures that are so important to the green of the canopy. The roots will also search out potassium and phosphorus when the tree decides to flower to produce nuts. The need for the bones will then be even greater. These are all matters of life and death to a tree and to a forest.

The microelements such as calcium, cobalt, gold, selenium and more come into play for enzyme control and regulation. These minerals are the universal catalysts found in trees and other plants, and in food. They are just as necessary to the human family and do the same things: regulate enzymes and control biochemical pathways. "Dem bones" fine-tune the workings of the tree, making it function like a well-oiled machine to furnish the planet with oxygen.

Wood Ash

Cheap gardening for the beginner . . .

I t will make your eyes water, so be careful. Save the wood ash from the grate of your woodstove, firepit, barbecue or fireplace. If this is unavailable to you, barter a plant, or an apple pie, for wood ash from someone you know. Store this wood ash in a metal container at the end of your garden or in a woodshed. Make sure there is a lid on it to keep it dry. An old metal dustbin will do the job perfectly. Now you have a treasure. It is free. It is an herbicide, a fungicide, an insecticide and a first-rate plant fertilizer.

The ash you are storing must be carefully kept dry at all times. It will last for about five years. Dry hardwood ash contains between 9 and 10 percent potassium hydroxide. In its dry state it is a form known as potassium hydrate. When you add water to it, the ash becomes potassium hydroxide, in a reaction that vents out heat. Its chemical formulation is KOH, the K being the potassium, a macronutrient for all plant life, and the OH making it dissolve easily into water and thus through rainwater into soils.

The pioneers carefully hoarded dried wood ash. They even built small stone houses in which to collect the ash safely away from the main house, just in case a live coal was amongst the ashes. These ash houses were in constant use, summer and winter. Dried ash was used as under-bedding for all animals. Then the straw was added. The floors of chicken houses were ashed, then the bedding laid down. This ash countered the strong effect of chicken manure when it was used out in the fields. All of the nesting boxes for laying hens received a handful of wood ash every week to keep lice away from the entire flock. An ash and lime sand bath in a tub was served up for the winter quarters of all fowl to keep the birds happy. Birds, wild and domesticated, enjoy a dust bath, which keeps their plumage healthy.

In the pioneer's home, wood ash was used as a lye solution, which is a potassium hydroxide solution of wood ash added to water. This lye was also called caustic potash because of its burning effect on the skin. Washing soaps, both hard and soft, were made by mixing lye with animal fat or tallow saved from cooking. Lye was also used to clean and whiten the famous elmwood tables of the countryside of Canada. This had the side effect of sterilizing the surface for food. Many children were set to scrubbing the floorboards using a lye wash and their mothers were judged accordingly.

Lye was and still is used all over the globe to rinse toxins out of food. For thousands of years the North American aboriginal peoples added lye to uncooked corn to remove the testa or outer, hard kernel coating to make hominy. The Mexican people also prepared maize in this way to make tortilla flour. The island cultures of the tropics used lye as a rinse to remove the neurotoxins from some of their fruits, nuts and spices before cooking with them.

In North America wood ash was used as a fertilizer, a brainchild of the aboriginal peoples. Wood ash was a perfect match for a climate that was dry during the summer months and damp in April and November. Natives maintained and controlled the great nut tree savannahs of eastern and central North America by setting flash fires in the spring and fall. These fires ran quickly, turning annual dry vegetation into a fine surface ash that fed the trees and acted as a pesticide targeting pathogenic insects.

There is another almost-lost history around wood ash. The global community used lye for washing tannins out of acorns. The white oak acorns are sweeter and require less lye than the red oak acorns. In the past, the acorn was a very important annual food. In parts of the Middle East and Asia, acorns are still sold in farmers' markets.

Gardeners can use wood ash to amend the soil. If the soil happens to be acidic, wood ash will sweeten the soil, bringing it into a range that is more suited to the majority of vegetables and flowering plants. If the soil happens to be alkaline, add a small amount of wood ash as a source of potassium fertilizer; a little in these circumstances will go a long way. My soil is alkaline. My vegetable garden is 20 by 36 metres (80 by 120 feet). I add about 10 litres (10 quarts) of wood ash peppered lightly across the soil in the spring and fall. This is the amount needed for flowering and successful fruiting.

Some perennials simply thrive when you sprinkle a cup of wood ash around the base of the plant in the first days of spring. These are all of the peonies, including the tree peony, carnations and pinks, all of the hellebores, hollyhocks, delphiniums, gypsophilas, clematis and roses. The ash helps with the flowering but also acts as an early fungicide on the surface of the soil, preventing the future development of black spot and mildews.

All the nut trees in my nuttery are ashed late in the fall, sometimes just before Christmas. These are the hickories, walnuts, filberts and butternuts. A litre (1 quart) of dried wood ash is flung around the base of the trees in a complete circle, catching the bark as far up as possible, and left to wash down the trunk in the next rain. The ash acts as a fungicide and an insecticide.

My entire orchard gets this treatment also, except that around 4 litres (8 quarts) are used for each tree. This ash is spread as a fine talc as far as the drip line of the tree where the canopy ends. The wood ash acts as a fungicide on the surface of the ground around the tree. Apples, pears, cherries, plums and apricots receive this ash in the early fall to penetrate the surface of the soil, deterring fungal spores.

In the early spring, Christian and I go on a tour of the bird boxes we have set up around the garden and orchard. It also involves a hike along our bluebird and tree swallow trail. We open the boxes from the bottom and scrape them out with a beehive tool. Then we fling a handful of dried wood ash into the bottom of the box. The birds build their new nests on top of this wood ash. It helps the nesting pair to remain healthy and free from feather parasites while they are tending to their young.

The wood ash in my barrel is precious. Treasures come and go. The beauty left behind in my garden is there forever with the sweet notes of the songbirds.

Lemon Love

Another way to protect your houseplants and garden . . .

Never call your cat Piano Toes. The fault was my daughter's. She noticed the six toes on the kitten in the shelter where we were picking out a new member of the household. On the way back home in the car she decided the cat's fate. He was to be named Piano Toes.

Then there was the first visit to my vet, James. He looked at the cat with its huge set of ears balanced by four paws, each with six toes. The kitten looked ridiculous, splaying itself out on the vet's metal table with its small miserable body under the parachutes of his ears. I never noticed his body markings then. They were too small and much too scrunched up. The design emerged months later.

James rested his two brown eyes on my new charge. I knew the meter of his disapproval before he uttered anything at all. "He's a runt. He won't amount to much. I suppose you want me to examine him. There is not much there to be examined. He's been starved." I put a hand on the kitten to protect him from further abuse. The animals in my household were studied, cared for, and well fed. James knew very clearly that I needed working cats in the garden and for the orchard because mice can do incredible winter damage to valuable and irreplaceable trees.

The following year I presented Piano Toes for his yearly roster of injections. "Got a new cat," James grunted, pulling out a tuberculin syringe from its paper coverings. "No," I answered, "that's the runt!" James put down the syringe and just stared at the cat. "Well, I'll be . . ." Piano Toes had turned into a 20-pound, black-and-white, Andy Warhol thing encouraging the use of the bullet on both sides of his body in perfect symmetry. Large and loud, a black bull's eye glared from each flank surrounded by black-and-white circles. The image had all the daring of Marilyn Monroe, staring down the viewer, focusing the audience into submission.

Piano Toes' feet rattled their tattoo of twenty-four nails on the sterling steel of the table. He had grown into his ears like a puppy. He proudly held his pinstriped business tail above his potential killing field. His coat glowed with health. He had joined forces with my dog, Finnegan's Wake, outside in the garden. They hunted together. The dog got the mice and the cat got the bunnies.

Inside my house, Piano Toes managed to turn my chesterfield into a large ball of rope. He then reduced the pine wainscoting by the kitchen door to toothpicks, arming the floor with deadly weapons. After Christian hastily replaced the wainscoting, Piano Toes repeated the shredding in half the time, his toes tingling with their workout and a smile on his face.

This cat was pushing me to extinction. So we faced off, the cat on one side and I the other. The cat had his cunning and I had my chemistry. Discoveries are only made by people on the margins. This is true of universities, where the top places of learning do not pop out inventions by the dozen. The real discoveries are made in smaller places by scientists using rubber bands and anything else that comes to hand. The same thing happened in my house. I came up with an idea. Lemons. Lemon love was the answer because it would not hurt the cat. It would teach Piano Toes a lesson in avoidance.

Lemons, limes, oranges, mandarins, citron and grapefruit all have a weapons capability. Just inside the rind there are circular land mines ready to go off. These are glands filled with volatile citrus oils. One dig of a fingernail into the skin to peel the fruit and the high-pressure trigger action is set off. Great shots of lemon, lime, orange and grapefruit fragrance ripple through the air. These are no ordinary smells. They are cannonballs of odour carried on the lift of other chemicals that readily disperse everywhere. If the site of landing happens to be the coat of a cat, the fur of a dog or even the feathers of a chicken, they will all flee to escape the phytotoxic chemical barrage. This is chemical warfare.

It becomes avoidance therapy when the citrus oil lands on the cat's fur. The cat must groom it off. Cats are clean, and it is their instinct to maintain their coat by licking off debris. So, if you want to protect a chesterfield, put a few oranges on the seat. If you want to protect an indoor potted plant, save some citrus peel and arrange it around the plant on the surface of the soil. Citrus scent works wonders for everything in the house that you want to cat- or dog-proof. And the animal is not harmed, just retrained by a chemical barrier.

White Cotton Shirt

If only the garden plants could wear one . . .

My garden is a kind of paradise in which I do my research. The garden itself is very large. It is composed of a fragrance border, a very large water garden, grapes, an orchard, a nuttery, the North American Medicine Walk and a vegetable garden divided in two by a huge hedge of Mary Washington asparagus. There is also a collection of rare and endangered trees dotted about everywhere to confuse matters.

My most recent research has been tracking down white cherries. White is a general term applied to cherries, because the colour can vary from pink to a dull crimson, the cherry holding a white cheek. These are the Bigarreau cherries, brought to Canada as seeds or seedlings by the early pioneers. They were grown in cherry orchards in this country by people who loved and cherished them. Now they have gone.

What is worse, they appear to have been lost, another tragedy for biodiversity.

A friend of mine was travelling the Alps. She knew that I had the white cherry on my wish list. Then a fluke happened, one of these instances when all you can do is be amazed at the coincidences of life. She noticed two very old cherries in a small alpine holding belonging to an elderly couple. The couple wanted to take down one of the trees. They were white cherries. She contacted me. I gave instructions for picking and preparing seeds for shipment. I grew trees from these white cherries that were added to my orchard last spring.

Christian and I do all the work in this garden. There is the pruning in the spring and the nut tree pruning, which happens in the late fall to minimize the bleeding of the sap. There is the collection, preparation, labelling and storage of seeds, carrying them over from year to year. Important species, such as the aboriginal bean collection, must be air-dried with moving warm air to prevent anthracnose setting into the new seeds. I look after the propagation of the rare species of small fruits, flowering plants, crosses and rare trees. All of this is over and above weeding and manuring.

In the last five years Christian and I have begun to wear white cotton as soon as the sun gets strong in the spring. It is not as easy as you would think to find plain white cotton shirts; we comb the stores for them. Usually we are left to trawl the charity stores and second-hand shops for what we want and most definitely need.

The shirts must be long sleeved with a good high collar. At the yoke, the back should have pleating to give the sleeves lots of room for movement. Usually I wear a man's shirt, several sizes too big for me, and Christian does the same. This is because we wear the shirts over our gardening clothes. The cheaper shirts are cotton, but sometimes a bargain can be picked up in linen.

Synthetic shirts are no good. The material off-gasses in the full sun. Cotton or linen are the best natural fibres. The weave matters also. Twill is superior, a complex weave of threads that are finely plied to form a fabric that is light, easy to wear, and will block out the sun.

Sun blocks are essential for gardeners or farmers or anybody who works out of doors during the summer months. An increase of carbon dioxide in the atmosphere acts like a wall for the bounce of high-energy waves of ultraviolet light. The greater the volume of carbon dioxide in the air, the more ultraviolet radiation will be bounced back to earth. This radiation can be increasingly felt on the surface of the skin as a prickly, hot sensation. Excessive exposure to UV light causes cancers like melanomas. Red-haired or blonde, light-skinned people are more easily damaged than dark-haired and dark-skinned people.

We try to do our more open work, like hoeing, in the early morning or later on in the afternoon. This is to avoid direct contact with UV. In the morning and evening the concentration of radiation is reduced. On some cloudy days, depending on the type of cloud cover, the concentrations, because of reflection, can be greater. Light clouds can increase this reflection. A heavy, dense cloud cover can block out much of the radiation. During heavy, overcast weather Christian and I will spend more time out in the garden than on sunny days. In spring and fall the UV radiation is less than in midsummer because of the position of the sun with respect to the earth.

White is a reflective colour. White acts as a foil for the body, reflecting the UV back into space. This colour, because it does not absorb the light, does not warm the body as black would. A black roof on a hot sunny day will get warm enough to fry an egg.

Sometimes I worry, now, about my plants. They sit in the soil, baking away in the sunshine. They do not have cotton shirts. Many are being forced to their wilt point by this intense reflected sunlight of recent years. It is a state of affairs in which the osmotic pressure disappears out of the two guard cells of each of the stomata or the mouth parts of the plants and the plant goes limp. I saw an awful lot of limp plants in the garden this past summer. But I live in hope and I am keeping my fingers crossed that you and I can stop this thing called global warming. It's down to us. Isn't it?

Perfect Lawn

A thing of the past. Get used to it . . .

In northern England, down a beech-lined avenue of mature trees, lies a walled garden. In the garden is a gardener. In the morning he applies sunscreen and leaves his shirt to flutter on a garden bench. He flexes his muscles doing calisthenics during lunch and tea break. Every day he manicures the perfect lawn. It is the correct shade of cooking-apple green, cut perfectly to within one inch of its life and crisply edged, the adjoining black earth a dark foil for the unity of the grass. When this grass grows, the gardener moves his Rolls-Royce mowing machine parallel to the edge of the lawn and begins cutting, moving the machine in careful rows. Then he criss-crosses the lawn again at right angles. There, within those four stone walls, lies the most perfect lawn in the world.

For two weeks every July the owner flies in from the United States to visit that lawn. He puts on a pair of bespoke English leather shoes over brown worsted stockings. A ruby ascot trims his houndstooth Harris tweed suit to a tee. He strides the lawn from end to end with a hunting crop in hand and an inspecting eye. Every blade of grass stands to attention. The gardener remains on the grey gravel path wearing his well-pressed Sunday suit, a white shirt and a purple and green tie. His head is bowed in respect, the cap almost tipping off his ample skull. When the inspection is over he sighs deeply. The lawn has passed the parade of yet another year.

The owner flies back to the Hamptons in his private jet. He returns to his life where time is judged by the hands of the stock market. And his money rolls around the world in hedge funds. His life goes on. His only pleasure, the perfect lawn, is an ocean away. He will see it, again, next year.

The rest of us have to settle for lawns invaded by weeds and quack grass. In spring, flashlights of dandelion and Bishop's weed rise to make a move when you least expect it. Ants make molehills and voles make anthills. The lawn mixture is never the correct one, some sewn for shade and the other for sun, both meeting unexpectedly to produce a bald patch. Then the Japanese beetles fly in at night, kamikaze-style, their offspring seeking grass roots for their supper. The lawn begins to float, turning into a wig of brown hair.

There is another way to make a perfect lawn. This one is cheap. It is easy to maintain. It does not require constant mowing. And, if the summer is dry, you do not need to pay a second mortgage in water bills to keep the grass growing. As an additional bonus, this lawn can be sat upon without fear of poisoning yourself, your family, your pets, your grandchildren and even your in-laws. This lawn does not need a daily haircut nor a gardener running a mower under your bedroom window before dawn.

In the springtime, which for most of the northern world is from February to April, and for the southern regions, from October to December, plant the bare patches in your lawn with any local hardy grass. Tamp the seed down by foot. Then buy a 1-kilogram (2.2-pound) bag of white-blossomed Dutch clover, whose seeds are small and round. The botanical name for it is *Trifolium repens.* With dry hands cast this seed all over your lawn. Go in a grid fashion, line after line, loosely spreading the seed. Then go at right angles to that, to get a complete covering of new seed on the grass lawn. If it is possible, roll the lawn. But this is not necessary. The first spring rains will wash the round seed into the soil.

White-blossomed Dutch clover will last in the lawn for a good fifty years. That kilogram of seed will cover 929 square metres (10,000 square feet) of lawn. Adjust the quantity of seed to the size of your lawn, though it does not matter if you broadcast too many seeds. The lawn will just be more luxurious.

The following day or so, spread one kilogram of ground dolomitic limestone over the freshly sown lawn. This will sweeten the soil, making way for the clover seed to catch or germinate. Once again, rain will wash this non-toxic fertilizer into the roots of the young grasses and clovers.

The limestone will last for over five years as a long-term fertilizer for both the grass and clover, establishing the roots. The Dutch clover, as it matures, develops special root bacteria that pull nitrogen out of the air and fix it into the plant. The clover in turn shares the nitrogen with the grasses so no more fertilizers are needed. This lawn is drought resistant and doesn't need watering. The little white clover blossoms feed honeybees and most of the beneficial insects. The insects stay around and go on to pollinate your vegetable garden and fruit trees, giving you a better, bumper crop of everything, for free.

Sit back. Enjoy your cheap lawn. It will be just perfect for your budget. Consider it to be your personal hedge fund, growing dividends for your future happiness.

Travel Thrombosis

A few tips to keep you healthy while you travel . . .

We have become a commuter society, but commuting is new to the human body. Legs were the locomotion of the past. Cars, trains, buses and planes may carry passengers safely on a daily basis but there is a hidden cost to be found inside the body of the commuter, invisible to the naked eye.

Global transportation makes use of many kinds of fossil fuels, most of which come from crude oil or natural gas extracted from the ground. There is one exception—Canadian tar sands produce crude bitumen oil. These crude oils are refined and pared down chemically to match the sophistication of the machine. Jets need highly refined oils whereas tractors can grunt away on diesel.

All these fuels are used the same way to move a tractor, truck or train: they are burned or combusted. The act of combustion tears apart the carbon bonding in fuel and releases the energy for propulsion. Each carbon finds a pair of oxygen molecules and carbon dioxide, a gas, is born. This gas flies off into the atmosphere to join its mates. Carbon dioxide is a heavy gas and carries debris with it as it is released from the car, train, bus or plane. This debris is a form of dangerous pollution, particulate pollution. It's invisible. The particles that are particularly nasty are those with a diameter of 2.5 microns or less.

This particulate pollution is about a third the size of a pollen grain and travels easily in the wind also. It becomes electrostatically charged and picks up passengers as hitchhikers. These are heavy metals like lead, chromium or arsenic. Sometimes some radioactive scouts can hitch a ride, particularly if there is warfare happening, anywhere in the globe. These radioactive travellers can be iodine, strontium or plutonium.

We breathe this invisible pollution into our lungs. It tracks its way into all the fine, feeding arterioles of the blood vessels of the body, forming inflammations that clog this network and reduce the ability of the circulation to do its vital work of gas exchange. This constriction pressures the heart by increasing blood pressure. Lungs, especially their lower regions, become clogged, too. Then we feel extremely tired and stressed.

To counteract these effects, all commuters should learn to relax at the end of the day. This relaxation should involve a walk around a garden, a treed street or a public park where there are grasses, flowers, trees and shrubs. The colour green is nature's balm, relaxing the body's nervous system and helping you to breathe more evenly and deeply. This in turn helps to empty the lower region of the lungs of their particulate pollution load. This green environment combined with deeper breathing helps to reduce the cortisol levels in the bloodstream, which triggers full-body relaxation, resting the adrenal glands and helping the kidneys. Once you have finished your walk, take a further five minutes over a cup of hot tisane. Even such a short respite helps the body recover.

Commuting by plane requires another set of tricks to stay healthy. Sitting for a long time in one given spot with the body strapped in place changes the flow characteristics of the blood itself. Blood is just a series of doughnut-shaped cells that move in the pipes of the circulation depending on the pressure exerted on them. If the flow rate of the blood slows, there is a chance that clotting can happen: a massing together of the doughnut cells because they have nowhere else to go. This is the medical condition called thrombosis, which can be fatal if that clot travels to the heart, brain or even the lungs.

A day or two before a plane trip, make sure you eat a meal with garlic in it. Garlic helps to move the doughnut cells along and to stop clotting. Finish that meal with an orange or two, which will help with the elasticity of the cell walls of the blood vessels and arteries. If you are fussy about garlic breath, eat a sprig of parsley to neutralize your mouth. And finally, when you fly remember to move a little, shifting your weight in the seat, wiggling your feet and if the flight is particularly long, taking off your shoes to exercise your legs. Get up and walk about the cabin.

Sometimes the horse and cart seems a far better way to travel.

Part III

The Larger World

Every time you take a step outside of your home
or office you are in the greater environment of
your life. That environment is shared with every
human being and creature of this planet. We are
all tied together in the living fold of nature.

In this section I want you to understand that
the trees on your own street improve your life.
And I want to tell you that the urban forest creates
a series of positive changes that can cause a powerful
waterfall effect in the city, ending with improved
social well-being, better health, increased property
values and a decrease in crime.

Each essay tells you something unique about the
world around us and lets you know that you have
a friendly tree nearby spilling out the very oxygen
that goes into each breath you take. At the very least,
a tree costs very little; at the very most, a tree will join

all other trees in sequestering carbon dioxide out of the atmosphere, abating global warming. Planting a tree or caring for one outside your front door on the street is something you can definitely do to help improve the greater environment in which we all live.

Winnipeg has an urban forest and it is a lesson to us all. The people look after their elms. They maintain banding around the trees to reduce Dutch elm disease. During the course of a foul winter, if the banding falls off, a Good Samaritan will replace it. The city glimmers green with the lush overhead canopies of these gentle giants.

Ottawa could follow suit, beginning with the gorgeous Parliament setting. I would suggest the catalpa. Then Toronto could follow, with Montreal, Regina, Calgary, Halifax and Vancouver—in fact, all of our cities and towns—joining in. Soon Canada would be in a league of its own, a jewel, with a setting no other country could match. Others would follow.

Planting Trees

If the Hells Angels can do it, so can you . . .

On the advent of the millennium I decided that I would do something to commemorate the year 2000. So I set about propagating twenty-two species of trees whose genetics were in decline in Canada. A good example is the bur oak, *Quercus macrocarpa*, the edible oak of Canada. Over the years of the pioneers settling the land, they always cut the best and straightest of these oaks to such an extent that the oaks that survived that onslaught became what's known to botanists as a retrograde species. Crooked and stunted bur oaks now dominate the landscape of our forests. I picked seed from an exceptionally straight and ancient oak from our own forest. Another tree I selected was the valuable Thomas walnut, *Juglans nigra* 'Thomasii.' (You can find a complete, annotated list of the species given out as our millennium project in the appendix.)

Christian and I put together three-quarters of a million seedlings and seeds of these selected varieties of trees. We paid for the project ourselves through plant sales of some of my unusual flowers. Some trees were sent off by express mail, bare root, to destinations in Canada and even the United States. We grew others to a good size in pots. (For two years, I sent out an SOS asking for plant pots that could be dropped off for me at the local library.) Some of the more rare species, like the wafer ash, *Ptelea trifoliata*, needed me to supply more than the usually printed planting instructions to willing participants: they needed to go to already competent gardeners and for me to follow up with expert advice. I asked everybody to report back to me on their progress and to ask for more advice if they needed it. We kept some seedlings and young trees here in the garden for our collection. It turned into the biggest tree planting ever launched in Canada by a private individual.

The idea was to set up epicentre forests, using the best genome possible, then to provide care and protection for these trees until they reached seed-bearing age. The pollen from these superior trees would spread and cross-pollinate locally, growing

trees to improve the entire breeding stock of the
native forests. Over time we could rebuild the
majestic forests of five hundred years ago.

All went well until the morning our garden was
to be open for interested local parties to come to
us directly to collect seeds or seedlings. I heard
motorbikes. A lot of motorbikes. The roadway to the
garden is half a mile long. The bikes kept coming.
I nearly collapsed when I saw a cascade of them swing
around the circle of the black walnut *allée* that leads
to the house. They were all in formation and in
black leather. Christian said, "It's the Hells Angels."
To say that my heart got stuck in my throat would
be an understatement. I think my increase in blood
pressure caused my hair to stand on end. It appeared
that they wanted Thomas black walnut trees. They
were going to do their bit. They had land in Ontario
somewhere. I will honestly admit that I did not ask
them where exactly. They received their nuts like
everybody else. They thanked me very graciously
for them and in perfect formation left the garden
proper with black leather, silver bits, fringes
and Hells Angels written on their backs, and
disappeared down the road again, leaving Christian

and me, silent, standing in a bath of gas fumes and road dust.

Schools and museums from both sides of the border asked for seeds. Many children were excited to begin a project that resulted in their own tree, which they treated like a pet. Housewives and mothers received seeds, and amateur and professional gardeners too. Business people came for trees to plant outside their buildings in the city. Farmers and landholders of all kinds received seeds. A group of wealthy women from Toronto waved blank cheques in my face, but the cheques were refused because my millennium project was free for all.

In the end, I can say that the trees were planted and well cared for. The children were downright delightful, charmed with the trees they saw growing and increasing in size in front of their eyes. Their moms and dads were equally pleased by the new connection to nature they saw in their children.

Before you plant a tree, look around. Gain some knowledge ahead of what you are about to do. Look and see if there is full sun or shade. Is the soil wet or dry? Imagine what changes come about if it rains. Will the site be swamped and waterlogged? Inspect the smaller plants around the spot you've chosen, the grasses, clovers and wildflowers. If they are having a tough time surviving, then the nutrition in the soil may require amendment. If they look green and lush, the soil is good. Generally if the soil is a dark, rich colour of chocolate with plenty of earthworms, it is a good soil and is excellent for growing anything. Trees are not too fussy; they will take their time if the soil is poor, but once they produce a canopy to shade the soil, they seriously get down to the business of growing.

All nut trees must have full sun for most of the day. They need it. The canopy has to have this sun so it can obtain sufficient photons to manufacture the flesh within the nut. A nut tree growing in the shade will starve. However, oaks will tolerate a little more shade. They can switch to producing one good acorn crop every two or three years to compensate for the lack of sun.

Following this principle, evergreen trees will survive in the shade because the canopy can capture and harvest photons of sunshine year-round except during the coldest days in the winter months. This allows the trees to stock up and keep surviving if

times get tough. These trees have modified leaves
to help them survive on dryer ground. Very few
Canadian trees, deciduous or evergreen, will survive
a waterlogged site, unless they are designed to do
so like the silver maple, *Acer saccharinum*, or the
tamarack, *Larix laricina*.

The next thing for you to do now is to pick up a
shovel. This is not a bad thing. You will get your
hands dirty. This will not damage you forever. Dig
a good-sized hole. Put your saved beef bones at the
bottom of the hole and step on them. Then put a layer
of soil on top. Take your tree very gently out of its pot.
Hang the tree in the hole to check where it needs to
sit so that it will be planted to the same depth that it
was in the pot or the nursery. Place the soil back into
the hole around the roots and tamp it down. Create
a saucer shape around the new planting about an
inch in height to catch water. Give your new tree
a thorough watering. Keep the soil damp for around
three weeks, which will give the tree time to generate
feeder roots.

I save and wash out milk cartons ahead of tree
planting. I cut and flatten the cartons, leaving a hole
for the trunk of the young tree. I arrange the carton

on the soil around the tree. The milk carton stops weeds from growing and shades the soil at the same time. This dual-purpose action helps the tree get an early start without the competition of weeds. It also cuts down on the amount of watering required. After a year or two I collect the cartons from the trees and begin mulching with cut grass.

This is how a modern forest is born—with intelligence and care. Trees get planted back into the ground along city streets and in suburban gardens, parks and public places. It started in Canada at the millennium. Now all we have to do is keep it going. If the Hells Angels understand that planting trees is necessary and can do it, so can you!

GREEN MACHINE

Learning to respect your local trees . . .

We have come a long way since the Middle Ages when the illegal cutting down of an oak tree carried a horrible punishment. The thief was shoved against a tree and his belly button nailed to the bark. He was then forced to walk around the tree in what soon turned into a death march. The 8.5 metres (28 feet) or so of his extended intestines ended up wrapped around the tree in a coil. The thief was left to die, slowly. Greed was not new then. It is definitely not new now. In fact, according to a report by Matthew Hansen in the *Proceedings of the National Academy of Sciences* in the United States, about 3 percent of the entire global forests that were standing in 2000 were gone by 2005. And nobody in the corporate world of the timber industry has lost a belly button.

In the past, members of a farming household had

more than a nodding acquaintance with trees.
Trees and forests were the backdrop of nature against
which the farmer plied his profession, that of putting
food on the table of others as well as on his own.
A good tree was like a prized heifer or a well-formed
foal. It represented value in itself and carried the
advantage of that value into the future. In other
words, capital and its direct offspring, interest on
that capital. This was of course green capital, for the
farmer works with the green machine.

The man who used to work our farm hit a wall in
the Dirty Thirties. He did not have, and could not
afford to buy, sufficient winter feed for his flock of
North Country Cheviot sheep. In the fall he released
them into the cedar woods behind his house and they
emerged from the winter looking well, their numbers
significantly increased by the birthing of lambs.
Later, he felled a prime tree for the local canal locks
to pay for an operation. Trees and the forest were his
insurance policy.

The seasons created by the green machine are
a timepiece for us all. Even in the city the early red
flowers of the maples against the bare bark of the
greying tree tell us that spring is on its way. Then in

summer comes the canopy, filtering sunshine and warding off the heat of a midday sun. Fall offers the riches of leaves to the compost that aids the soil's renewal; all seems well and settled for the big sleep of winter. The short days sharpen shadows that climb into unexpected places and soon we hope again for the lengthening days of spring.

In North America the aboriginal world watched the white oak, carefully noting the changes in the little, brown, dry winter tips of the branches for their first greening. This lime-green signal was the seasonal clock they used for planting the corn that was a staple for millennia. The oak is finely tuned to the solar heat of the sun, requiring exactly the same BTU, or thermal units, that the corn seed must have to germinate and grow to maturity.

The trees of the Americas were like the trees of the rest of the globe: the fat baobabs of Madagascar and Australia, the towering eucalyptus of the Eden of Tasmania, the pines of Greece and Spain, the stout oaks of Europe, the medicinal miracle trees of the boreal forest system and the sugi of Japan. They represent food, shelter and medicines. Most seniors living today remember being caught out in a shower

of rain as a child, and running to the nearest tree
to flatten their body against the trunk to stay dry.
The rain or shower lashed through the canopy, but
somehow the child, snuggled against the trunk,
remained dry. And then there was that moment of
waiting and watching for the rain to go in a sylvan
silence that drove an understanding of nature deep
into the consciousness of the child, a memory that
was a harmonic ending to the song of the rain. We
carry those notes of silence forever.

We need to look up with respect at trees and what
they do for us as companion species and what they do
for the health of the planet. Like the farmers of old,
we should remember that the trees and global forests
are the backdrop of nature, the only one working for
us. They are the molecular memo, harvesting one
carbon atom at a time, by which we put food on the
table, plate by plate, cup by cup and spoonful by
spoonful. And they pulse that sweet gas we call
oxygen, needed for every single breath we take,
using the regulation of special cells.

The green machine runs the tapestry of nature,
fired by the sun's fuel in the green of all plants
everywhere. Your own local tree is a cog in that

machine. Protect it. That tree is part of the green molecular machinery of the global forest system, which is the common inheritance of our human family, carving out a future for us all.

CITY FORESTS

More trees in cities, please . . .

A city is an art form. Major cities represent the collective design ability of a nation expressed in buildings, a form of geometric literacy. Capital cities reflect the desires, wishes and hopes of a people, set in stone, concrete and wood. The impact is a word we call culture, with a flavouring of east or west together with a peppering of religion in the multi-coloured dish of global humanity.

But without the tree a city is as dead as a statue. Trees have come out of the workbox of nature as the best that can be produced. They are works of art based on a rule of dichotomy, the division of one into two. This is the simplest and most elegant of forms in art, based on mathematics. The dichotomy of division produces the pattern language of nature that spells out the tree from one single seed into a powerful living creature.

Trees are important to cities because cities are congested. People live closely together in small spaces. The modern cars, trucks, buses, trains and planes add their fumes. The atmosphere of a city is always smoggy. It is visible in summer as a sheet of haze over the heart of the city caused by a lift in rising air with the heating effect of the sun. Sometimes that smog rides the air over the city, giving us smog days lasting for long stretches of the summer. The geography of the landscape can make smog worse especially if the city sits in a valley, like Mexico City. The air can never really clean itself.

City forests help to abate smog-laden air. Trees during daylight hours are prodigious oxygenators. They oxygenate the city air, lightening it, because oxygen is a much lighter gas that helps to dissipate smog. The molecular form of oxygen is very stable and as it moves upward in the city atmosphere it helps to separate smog, dispersing it.

Trees, in the presence of sunlight, move and orient the leaves of their canopy to harvest the atmosphere. Trees need carbon dioxide, which is a toxic gas produced by congestion and the combustion of traffic. The busier the city streets, the more active the leaves. Carbon dioxide from the lungs of people and from petroleum products is a food that really matters to trees. They can split this gas up into carbon and oxygen, but it is really the carbon that they crave. Trees take this carbon, atom by atom, and build it up into their body. A carbon atom breathed out by your child in the early morning can become a carbon atom belonging to the tree by noon.

The less toxic parts of smog or pollution are also of interest to a tree's digestion. A tree can comb the air and reduce the pollution. The leaves of many trees have microscopic features, either on the upper part of the leaf or on the lower part, that act like the fine teeth of a comb. These are called leaf hairs. Sometimes these hairs are glandular, holding oils and resins; then they are called glandular hairs or trichoma. Collectively all these hairs comb the atmosphere of pollution, big and small.

Tiny pollution particles lodge in the valleys of the leaf's surface between the hairs. But the leaf has another trick to remove them. The floor of these valleys, called a cuticle, is like linoleum. It has a waxed finish. This floor does not like to hold water because it is waxed. Rain and mists wash off the leaves very easily, carrying all the pollutants with it. Sometimes they are in solution and other times, they are just carried along in a microscopic tsunami down the trunk.

The trunks of trees, too, help with the flow of water, because they are usually fissured and crazed. They direct the rainwater to the base of the tree where the soil will happily soak it up and move it along. The pollution gets separated from the rainwater by the chemical and physical character of the soil that is like a sieve. Much of the pollution gets trapped at or near the surface of the soil around the root system of the tree, which also helps to widen the dispersal of the water. The tree is still not finished with the pollution, not by a long shot. Pollution in the atmosphere is just another word for tree food.

The best part of a tree is invisible. It is the underground root zone, usually about one-third the size of the canopy; if the canopy is large the roots are too. Some roots take a dive into the soil and are called the taproots. Others spread out along the soil or just underneath it; they are called adventitious roots. They all work to feed the tree.

The underground zone of the tree is a metropolis. There is a network of bacteria and fungi working together to form a feeding and delivery frenzy with the root hairs of the trees. This is called the mycorrhiza. The network of the mycorrhiza takes the pollution out of the rainwater in the soil and recycles it down to a molecular level. These microscopic creatures of the soil with bare-bones-DNA work like a hive of hungry bees armed with enzyme tools to split apart and rejoin everything coming their way.

The mycorrhiza runs a co-op with the roots of the tree. It is a very satisfactory relationship that has stood the test of time, approximately 400 million years. The soil bacteria and fungi need sugars produced by trees and the tree needs the recycled minerals from the pollution products reworked by the microbes. An exchange takes place. The mycorrhiza use the sugars for the energy to retool the enzymes for minerals and metals needed by the tree. With the aid of the minerals and metals, the tree grows a bigger canopy and a better root system, which helps the microbes of the mycorrhiza to multiply. Everybody benefits.

All of the tree's underground system of traffic is, in turn, regulated and restructured by a microscopic creature called a bacteriophage. They have just been discovered in the past ten or so years. Knowledge of the bacteriophage is still a work in progress by scientists and will be for a long time yet. The bacteriophage population breaks and remakes the soil bacteria and fungi. Sometimes they digest them and rework them into antibiotics or fungicidal and anti-viral molecules, especially if it looks like the tree is becoming sick. The message sent by the tree to its roots is a chemical one based on phenols. The bacteriophages listen to this message and do a quick whip-about, producing temporary medicine to help the tree fight off the sickness. They exist in the soil and in the sea, also. It has come as a surprise to the scientific world that bacteriophages are the most numerous creatures on the planet. They are the subordinate army of the tree.

In a city, a tree or a forest is beneficial. The tree is the most highly evolved creature of the plant kingdom. It donates oxygen to feed the human brain, molecule by molecule, and breath by breath. So we need more trees in cities . . . please.

Unexpected Benefits

Urban trees can stop urban crime . . .

She was hiding from the horrors of middle age
with a pretty coral-coloured cashmere shawl.
She was appointed as my aide-de-camp by the
university authorities. My public lecture, social
and media events in Toronto needed a personal
touch. She was there to guide me through the rigours
of traffic in a city that has forgotten to sleep.

Over early morning Irish breakfast tea, her
brown eyes told me she was in deep trouble. As
her hand held her cup, it trembled a little. Her
husband had just announced that he was leaving
her. It was a planned exit, with the sale of their
country house to the north and their city condo,
too. He divided the booty down the middle. He
had pulled up his anchor to set sail, unfurling his
testicles for the islands of youth with his sack of
money and a very bald head.

She was left hanging on to her principles in this shipwreck of a life. She loved the city and desperately wanted it to have a future. She was worried about the environment and she did not want her grandchildren to grow up with drugs and crime as constant companions. She understood the connections out there on the city streets. She recycled and watched her carbon footprint, going down to the St. Lawrence Market to buy local food. She desperately wanted to make a difference, to do something that improved the lot of others. Then she asked me the simple question: What could she, a single individual, do to help nature?

I told her to bring nature back into the city in the form of the urban tree. It is simple and cheap. Plant a tree and then care for it, an easy thing for anybody to do. A tree is an investment in yourself and your future. Trees are living creatures. On streets they breathe a form of liberty and democracy, because everybody can enjoy a tree. In a city park, where people can sit and relax together, trees build community. Trees bring out the more social aspects of the human family and because they do this, crime, especially urban crime, has been shown to be reduced in a treed location.

There are many good reasons to plant an urban tree. Urban trees reach out and into the carbon dioxide–laden air of the streets. This air has a long shelf life if it is left alone. A tree sequesters this gas in the skeletal wood of its body by way of the leaves. Populations who live and play in such carbon dioxide–laden air have a diminished reasoning capacity. The tree spills oxygen as a byproduct of photosynthesis into the urban area, increasing the capacity of the brain through an increased oxygenation of the blood, which turns on the tap of intelligence and health.

Shopkeepers and merchants should have a direct interest in the urban tree in front of their store. The presence of green foliage seems to loosen the purse strings, and spending in these relaxed areas goes up by about 9 percent, according to studies done in the United States. They are confirmed by research in England, also, by Neville Fay of Treework Environmental Practice. The growing body of work of the Ontario Urban Forest Council and Tree Canada helps support the evidence of the importance of urban trees.

There is another good reason to plant an urban tree. Urban trees improve overall health, thus

reducing the cost of health care. The space under
a large green canopy of elm or maple on a hot, muggy,
humid day is 25 percent less polluted. The tree cleans
the airborne dandruff and maintains a cleaner space
underneath the canopy. This helps children with
asthma and people who suffer from breathing
problems, as well as those with heart disease.

A good-sized urban tree like a bur oak or any white
oak will reduce the damaging effects of ultraviolet
light on the skin, decreasing the incidence of skin
melanomas. The oak produces its own sunscreen
called quercetin that has a dissipating effect on
ultraviolet light. This high-energy light has the
ability over time to cause considerable damage to
painted surfaces, bleaching them and even the
aluminum and concrete fabric of buildings. Shade
on buildings reduces these expenses considerably.
Shade on the urban home saves on curtain, carpet
and even furniture-fabric replacement. Paintings,
oils or watercolours, are seriously damaged by being
exposed to increased UV light, as many art galleries
have found to their great cost.

The urban tree does something that is invisible to
the naked eye: it changes the humidity index of the

air. A mature tree transpires, drawing the moisture out of the soil through its plumbing system and releasing it at the surface of the leaf. This flow of moisture is felt in the air as humidity. In addition, the anatomy of a tree is built like a condenser unit, with the outside of the tree relatively waterproof. So the tree can catch the moisture of the morning dew and shed it down the tree. This, too, adds to the humidity. Air that is humid is easier to breathe and is a softer force on the surface of the lungs.

In times of drought, the shade of a tree buys around three weeks' worth of savings in watering. This is important to the budget of city managers who maintain green spaces and public parks within a city. Water shortages have become more acute in recent years for cities with large populations. Shade helps considerably.

Many groups are now in the process of planting an edible landscape within cities, Ottawa being one example. These are urban trees that bear fruits like apples and pears together with nuts from North American native trees like the kingnut, edible acorns and butternuts. These foods are free for the public. And, of course, they add to the menu for birds and butterflies.

Urban trees as edible landscapes are community builders and boosters. A strong community is a safety net, the only one, for people who are disenfranchised. It is another route away from crime and toward safer cities, especially for the young. A little urban tree can teach an enormous lesson in the classroom of a city.

ANTI-CANCER TREES

The secret medicines of trees . . .

Different cultures produce different philosophies toward disease and therefore multiple treatment possibilities. The ancient Celts used prescriptive medicines long before the birth of Christ. Some, like mistletoe, *Viscum album*, are still in use today as a fermented extract called the Iscador treatment for solid tumours. The epiphyte of choice was the mistletoe from the oak, *Quercus robur*, and not from the apple, *Malus*.

North American aboriginal medicine men and Tibetan healers both used a form of dreaming to obtain a plant cure. They believed each plant had a life force or spirit but that the spirit of the plant would reveal its medicine only when needed. During the process of deep meditation, they would ask the species to reveal its healing secret.

Around 60 percent of all the medicines in use today come from a plant source. Some species of trees like the yew, *Taxus brevifolia*, produce medicines that are too complex to copy. These are paclitaxels, used in the treatment of cancer. The atoms are arranged in the molecule in three dimensions, like the walls of a house, though the walls move and switch places, and then rotate upside down when used as a key to unlock a cell. A plant that produces the similarly complex chemical taxodione, which also exhibits extraordinary spacial geometry, is the sacred tree of Japan, the sugi, *Cryptomeria japonica*, long considered to be a healing tree.

All around the world and even at your own doorstep there are trees that hold incredible medicines waiting to be unlocked. Some of them have been known or suspected for a long time and appear in folk medicines. Others are part of the oral culture from Arab, Greek or Roman thinking. Even the Chaldeans, who were an ancient Semitic people of Babylonia, used a tree onion, *Allium proliferum*, for its medicine, whose molecules are currently under investigation in laboratories as shields to prevent cancer growth. This onion is not a tree, though, even if it does grow a little like one. It is in the onion family.

The more common species of anti-cancer trees for the North American continent are the redwoods, representatives of the *Taxodiaceae* family, and all of the yews of the *Taxaceae* family. We have the rue or *Rutaceae* family whose fruit, oranges, limes and lemons, are common to the kitchen and the entire birch or *Betulaceae* family, which includes the delicious hazelnut. We shouldn't forget the oaks, all of them, or the beech or *Fagaceae* family and of course the walnut, *Juglandaceae*, whose member, the black walnut, has leaves filled with the lemon scent of ellagic acid, which shields the entire body from cancers, as does eating the nuts. The *Annonaceae*, or custard-apple family, produces a fruit, the Canadian pawpaw, that is also streaming out many anti-cancer possibilities in our laboratories today.

Like humans, the tree has evolved over time to be the kingpin species in the world of plants. A tree has extremely complex DNA, only different from the human kind by two bases, the overall size of the tree's DNA being greater. The tree produces its array of medicine for its own protection. It is incumbent on the tree, if it is to survive and reproduce, to be smart.

Like the human body, the tree is covered by a continuous skin. On us it is the epidermis, on the tree it is the cambium, protected by the bark. Underneath the bark, the square, solid, cambium cells hum with life. They are the brainy matter of the tree. To kill a tree, cut the cambium in a circle around the trunk and the tree will die. Porcupines do this by default to get at the rich, protein-packed nutrition of the cambium cells, which they love.

Medicines are produced in the cambium cells, but the amounts differ depending on the tree's exposure to the sun. The areas of the bark to the south should have more medicine than the bark with a northern exposure. Tree medicines are transported to the roots also. But the leaves, as they mature into the growing season, manufacture and sometimes retain the largest supply. The leaf of a tree is the factory of a tree. The leaf has distinct tissues that function like different organs in the body.

The leaf has a window-like cuticle on the surface that lets in light to a green organ beneath it called the mesophyll. The mesophyll is made up of an arrangement of sacs. Each sac is called a chloroplast.

Inside the chloroplastic sac lie the solar energy receptive molecules called chlorophyll. The chlorophyll catches the photons from sunshine and transfers this moving sunbeam into chemical building blocks. Some of these blocks become medicines for the tree's health and welfare. They, in turn, become medicines for people.

Many of these tree medicines are aerosols. Others are moved around the tree by the transport system of the tree's vascular abilities, much like human circulation. Some medicines are reworked into killer compounds for other plants called allelochemicals, and are released either into the wood of the tree or as water-soluble leachate into the soil. More again are refined into a super-soluble form and released into the water as aldehydes, destined for streams, lakes and rivers. Other trees are prone to infections from endogenous fungi and produce their own chemicals to control fungal growth so the fungus doesn't take over.

Probably the most interesting medicines are the aerosols, which the human eye can see as a blue haze over a distant wooded area. Closer up, we inhale them as a perfume or odour of some kind. The mechanism to lift these chemicals into the air and release them into a form where they are propelled by air movement is much the same as NASA's Apollo system, except it happens on a molecular level. The boost is given and two molecules are on their way; one falls off and the last one flies as an aerosol medicine around the airways of the forest and into the atmosphere.

When the tree decides to launch its medicinal aerosol load, it releases the aerosol from the little green sacs of the mesophyll into the air spaces between the sacs. The aerosols gather at the mouths of the leaves for release, often triggered by the humidity index of the surrounding atmosphere, coupled by an increase of temperature. The two guard cells, one at each side of the mouth, or stoma, go flaccid. The aerosols are released with the lips' opening. On a hot, humid, sunny day the atmosphere around the trees of the forest is filled with medicinal aerosols.

The Japanese frequent their fragrant forests of sugi and yew on a sunny day, walking, sitting or just enjoying nature as it unfolds around them. The aerosols flood the air and bathe every part of the body, the skin, the mouth, the nasal passages and even the lungs with medicinal molecules. The

Japanese call this process forest bathing: a sophisticated way of taking one's medicine to improve health.

Forest bathing is taking off in North America, too, and about time.

The Power of Pawpaw

The most important tree nobody has heard of . . .

Let me rant for a moment. Botanically speaking, the pawpaw, *Asimina triloba*, is one of the most important trees of Canada. Yet few have heard of this species, let alone seen it. Toronto sits on its native habitat. Long before that sprawl of buildings and roadways, these little trees used to live in the heat sinks of sandy banks looking out to Lake Ontario.

The pawpaw has other siblings in the tropics, some in Central America or Brazil. The best grow in the tropical highlands of the Andes in Peru. In fact, archeological digs in Peru regularly expose the bean-like seeds in prehistoric remains. These are almost always the seeds of the cherimoya, *Annona cherimola*, a delicious, heart-shaped, green fruit whose custard filling tastes heavenly, like a mixture of pineapple with mango and bananas. The Toronto baby is just as sweet and delectable.

The ripe fruit tastes so good but it is known only to raccoons, opossums and many other four-legged animals. They have a shopping list with the pawpaw as the number one fruit to eat at all costs. They are a slave to the taste of the fruit, so much so that the genetics of the tree began to depend on them for dispersal. This began a long time ago, perhaps thousands, maybe even millions of years ago.

When I got the seeds of the pawpaw from a region south of Toronto, I knew I had a problem. The beans are extremely difficult to germinate and to grow. I wanted to plant this tree in my North American Medicine Walk, an area of the garden where I collect the ancient medicines of continental North America. I had the idea that I would grow and then propagate this species so other botanical gardens would have it, too.

One day, I cracked the problem of germination. I was sitting quietly by the water garden when a female raccoon came to drink. She had a handful of black cap raspberries in her paw and she turned them over and over. I never realized that these creatures were so agile and dexterous. They have to be seen in action to be believed. I had a flash of inspiration. I will not say genius, because it was such a little thing. I had the answer, though.

All creatures produce oil to keep their skins supple, and raccoons, which I knew to be crucial to the propagation of pawpaw trees, have oily paws. The fruit's seeds are large enough to become a worry bead for a raccoon. In the process of handling the seed, sebaceous oil is transferred to the seed coat or testa. The oil seals the outer coat so that no oxygen can get in. This seal closes off the embryo inside, maintaining a full dormancy, which slowly changes as the oil wears off during the winter months. A time-release capsule! Copying the action of the raccoon, I got my pawpaw seeds, wiped the side of my nose, and rubbed the nose grease onto the seeds. In due course I successfully germinated them. I planted my trees.

The flowers of the pawpaw are a deep blood brown ranging to black. Most species are primitive and reluctant to be fertilized. The male part of the flower produces pollen that is always too late to be received by the stigmas of the female reproductive organ, so the flowers rely on insects or beetles to cross-pollinate them. Hand pollination has been practiced for a long time in the Andean valleys, but the Canadian *Asimina triloba* flower seems to set fruit in a normal manner. The fruit has a fleshy inside like a soft apple in which the seeds are embedded. The green 3- to 5-inch fruit turns brown as it ripens into the fall. The best fruit has a yellower soft custard filling, giving the species another name, the custard apple.

The aboriginal peoples throughout the Americas knew the custard apple. It was a special fruit for them to eat in the late fall. The Hopi peoples loved it, calling it the frost banana in their language. There was also a ritualistic hunt for this fruit that is still carried out today in regions of the Appalachians where the flesh is saved for cooking or frozen for the winter months and made into ice creams, sherbets and pawpaw flump, a meringue made from sugar beaten into pawpaw flesh and folded into egg whites.

The pawpaw tree is small, growing to 9 metres (30 feet). It will not stand waterlogged roots, which will kill it, nor temperatures of -40°C (-40°F). Super-cold nights will reduce its growth with such damage that it will not thrive. Well-drained sandy soil, with a windbreak of a bank acting as a heat source facing due south and also, if possible, facing a source of water for extra solar reflection, is the ideal habitat for this tree. In this situation, our northern pawpaw will be able to manufacture some truly remarkable medicines that go into the yellow flesh of the fruit.

These medicines are a family of biochemicals called acetogenins. So far 250 separate biochemicals have been characterized at the University of Kentucky, all new to science. What is unusual about these molecules is that they are fat soluble and appear to have the ability to unplug an essential enzyme called nicotinamide adenine dinucleotide (NAD) in a tumour cell, which means that a cancerous cell becomes marooned in the body without a power source to make it multiply. It is like a stalled car with an empty petrol tank.

The pawpaw offers another means of arresting the growth of cancer, one that can enter the fat tissue of the body and do its work. It also shows promise in the treatment of malaria and other parasitic infections. My little nose-grease experiment shows that the tree can be grown by the human hand. The seeds can be obtained from trees growing in the wild on the northern shores of Lake Erie. The Canadian pawpaw will produce the best medicine, because it grows on the margins and therefore has the strongest immune system. It can be the basis of a new food and used as a fragrance in the cosmetics industry, too.

Let me finish my rant. My nose tells me that the pawpaw should be saved. By Canadians. For more reasons than just one.

MONEY TREES

Mother Earth banks carbon, not gold . . .

The biblical Eve told her children that money did not grow on trees. And since then, every mom and dad has warned their sons or daughters of the very same thing.

They were all wrong, every single generation since the caveman put down his club to hitch up his loincloth. Money does grow on trees, because trees are money.

Mother Nature produces wealth beyond all understanding. Her timeline has been long in the perfection of her product, millions upon millions of years of painstaking research with absolute quality control at the end of it. The rejects die. Her projections are exponential in growth, a guarantee of customer satisfaction. Her stores are expansive but not endless. Her ingenuity is infinite. She was on a roll up to a few centuries ago.

Mother Nature uses the carbon standard instead of the gold one. She began this banking system shortly after her rather rocky birth. She sources this carbon from the great pool of the atmosphere and banks it in trees. She taps the sun to do the specialized welding job needed for this, using photons that are spit out by the sun's tremendous heat. The carbon is cut out of the atmospheric gas, carbon dioxide, at a rate of one carbon atom per one molecule of gas. Then this carbon is added into the trees, like little black atomic pearls, one at a time. They grow into forests.

Forests are the carbon reserves of nature, banked into a living system that multiplies with its own wealth. Forests also experience death. The carbon remains. It goes back into storage in the form of underground vaults. This fossilized carbon re-emerges from time and pressure as diamonds, coal and turf. It also liquefies while still in underground storage as oil or as the gas methyl hydride.

The forest banks of nature provide services to their clients who come in through the sun-polished doors of the carbon cathedrals. These services include the production of oxygen, a life-giving, atmospheric gas required by every breathing creature on this planet.

There is also the continuing sequestration of carbon out of the atmosphere, rendering the atmospheric gas mixture a safe one to breathe. The forests provide food, medicine and phytochemicals. The terpenoid aerosols released by forests govern the weather patterns of land, sea and air. The leachates from forests manage the micronutrient iron levels in saltwater, which is a nighttime signal for growth and the foundation feeding for the entire ocean. Another service is planetary cooling and infrared reflection. Then, of course, there is the atmospheric scrubber or detergent effect of the antibiotics, fungicides and antivirals released on a daily basis, which are the ecological shields of a living planet. The forest also has a special value-added product in timber and wood. On top of this, forests maintain potable fresh water by filtration and convection all over the global landscape.

The holdings of Mother Nature's bank are diverse. They are all trees, of course, each one represented by the unique qualities of a different family. Some families prefer the spectacular cold of the boreal and will not settle for anything less. Others love the tropics, frugal leaf-huggers who hate the cold. And then there are the in-between temperate trees that move north when the mood suits them. Their market is a truly global one, because forests occur on all continents and islands, from the edge of the Arctic to the tips of South America, Africa, Asia, Australia and New Zealand.

One tree with an edge on the North American banking system is the black walnut, *Juglans nigra*. A well-grown, mature tree can fetch $60,000 at auction. This is because the wood is rare, dark and stable, good for creating veneer, and is even medicinal. It also off-gasses small amounts of juglone as a fungicide. Unfortunately, it can only be grown successfully in North America because the canopy needs the higher solar exposure produced by the profile of this continent.

Another tree with an edge, this time in Europe, is the common English oak, *Quercus robur*. The wine industry, whose vineyards are expanding with the warmer weather and better growing conditions for the grape, needs oak in a very big way because oak is the ideal storage vehicle.

Another tree that does not punish the purse to grow from seed is the matumi or Transvaal teak, *Breonadia salicina*. The African sun fills this protected tree with treasure, an oil that is an insecticide, naturally protecting the wood from termites. The lustre of this polished hardwood carries flame-like markings that make it the darling of cabinetmakers worldwide.

The baobab of continental Africa, Madagascar and Australia is an aboveground storage tank for water, which should have a greater value than oil, for water will quench the thirst in growing heat. Fresh water is stored in this tree in its spongy parenchyma tissue, whose osmotic pressure holds this enormous tub of a tree together. Scientists, particularly physicists, cannot understand how the tree does it.

There is also a sacred tree with clever connections to the gods of India, the banyan. This moving monster is a Bengal fig, going by the name of *Ficus benghalensis*. This tree "walks" by means of giant aerial roots and produces a canopy that can shade acres of ground. Shade from the killing heat is the great gift to India and this epiphytic tree accomplishes this task in spades.

Then there are the silk cotton trees, *Ceiba pentandra*, or kapok-bearing trees of South America. These giants of the tropics produce large seedpods filled with light brown hairs that make an ideal natural insulator or stuffing for furniture, bedding and sleeping bags. Commercially, these trees are a gold mine.

The trees of the carbon castle of Mother Nature are capable of laying down another framework for a green economy. It will be based on a global banking system that has been a blockbuster in the past, offering carbon credits to sustain our future. Now all we need is the foresight and perseverance to grow forests and money trees.

Bog Birch

The boreal birch will make you sleek and slim . . .

O ver the years I have steadily worked at repatriat-
ing North American plants back to Canada.
Sometimes I fail to find the species I'm looking for,
and fear that it is lost forever. Other times I succeed
by cunning. The owners of the great houses of Ireland
and England had sticky fingers when it came to
stocking their gardens. The late Ambrose Congreve
created a magnificent plantation of the cucumber
tree, *Magnolia acuminata*, in his 34-hectare (84-acre)
manicured garden, Mount Congreve, in Ireland. He
only knew that they were the correct species for sure
when I confirmed this in his garden, since I grow
them, also. With such expert advice and confirma-
tions, over the years, I have bartered with botanical
hoarders for my choice of rare and unusual seeds.

My great interests are species holding cures to
cancer, immune system boosters and cardiotonics

of various kinds. Currently, I am establishing a
repository of these species for the future, since
there are no private botanical research gardens in
Canada doing this. In addition, I am interested in
the nutritional aspects of North American nut trees.
The aboriginal peoples called them anti-famine
trees. I cross and breed these trees for their improved
food value and flavour, and for the gains in health
they offer into the daily menu.

One fall day a little seed caught my eye. It was
a tiny one with two small wings. The belly of the seed
bordered by the wings looked as if it would explode
with the effort of remaining dormant. It was a seed
on offer by the Irish Garden Plant Society (IGPS),
from one of the main country house estates of
Ireland. The seed was from a tiny tree they had
growing in a rockery. The tiny tot was a true-blue
Canadian. I wanted it.

The tree in question was a bog birch bearing
the name of *Betula pumila* var. *glandulifera*. How it
arrived in Ireland from the Canadian Arctic or from
Newfoundland, I have no idea. It must have happened
centuries ago when the firstborn son inherited the
estate and title. The other sons were either turned

into clerics or globetrotters who returned home with
seeds or parrots in their pockets just in time to gather
up their allowances and/or brides, before setting off
on their travels again.

The bog birch is a slender little tree with fuzzy
leaves that looks more like a bent-over shrub than
a tree. This form expresses itself beautifully in the
design of a rock garden. The leaves wear a fur coat
of brown hairs to protect them from the bitter cold of
the arctic winter. Each hair is a gland that produces
an oil known as birch oil, which gives the entire tree
its sweet and fragrant smell. The bog birch goes
overboard protecting itself against the cold. Even the
male, pollen-bearing catkins and the small, rounded,
brown, woolly, female catkins produce a protective oil.

The bog birch is a Canadian boreal forest species.
The Chipewyan and Slave nations have used it as
a medicine for millennia because it is a member
of one of the most important medicinal families,
Betulaceae, of the north. A refreshing tea or tisane
can be made by brewing fresh leaves and little pieces
of stems obtained from the tops of branches in
boiling water. This brew is allowed to steep and is
consumed as it cools. This tisane helps to trim the

body of excess weight and it is drunk for that purpose. It helps to improve the circulation, relieve joint pain and decrease the effects of diabetes. This birch tea should also be enjoyed for the aroma of its aerosols, liberated in the form of a mini steam bath for the nose and lungs.

There are three chemical sisters in the bog birch: betulin, betulinic acid and methyl salicylate. In addition, there is a dwarfing compound called a gibbane biochemical that is found in every cell of this tree, acting as a phytoregulator, maintaining the dwarfed shape as a form of protection against intense cold. All four biochemicals act together as a mild medicine when drunk in a tisane, along with another biochemical, betulafolienetriol, which is active as an antibiotic against a particularly modern mugger, *Staphylococcus aureus*, a bacterium whose populations are on the rise in our modern world.

The betulin is a precursor to betulinic acid, a potent medicine if ever there was one. This acid induces apoptosis, or cell suicide, in human melanoma cells, in a form of tumour-cell-specific cytotoxicity. It holds high therapeutic potential. The research on betulinic acid is worldwide. Some of this research also shows that betulinic acid seems to inhibit HIV replication. The painkiller methyl salicylate is similar to Aspirin, the most ubiquitous drug ever used in pain management.

The dwarfing compound, the gibbane biochemical, is of particular interest to me. It is the nucleus of a plant-growth hormone isolated in 1938 from a fungus that caused a disease in rice. Since then this nucleus has been found everywhere in the plant kingdom. It is responsible for each flower that opens and is pollinated, producing our food. In addition, the gibbane is responsible for the growth response in plants with respect to soft sounds, like the human voice, maybe even birdsong. The ancient art of singing while sowing crops does have a positive and measurable effect on the final harvest.

The bog birch would be an ideal tree for an urban setting as a medicinal aerosol producer for the family and home. It would fit very well into a tiny garden. The fragrant foliage would only add to the enjoyment of the green space and act as a mild antibiotic, a natural one, to help keep growing children infection-free.

The bog birch from the Canadian north should be grouped into threes for visual effect in design and planted into hospital gardens as part of a garden bioplan to help in the healing of cancer patients, especially those with prostate cancer, against which betulinic acid appears to be particularly effective. It would cost very little and the gain would be great.

This bog birch is a small and humble Canadian tree bearing gifts from the boreal for us and for the entire planet.

Haw Trees

The hawthorn is a magical tree . . .

The sweet smell of jasmine is one of my favourite perfumes in the garden. Yellow jasmine, *Jasminum mesnyi*, is an evergreen climbing vine that should be grown under glass. It is delicate, trailing, and the flowers seem to gush out an invitation to pick. At least, that is how I read the situation as a child in Ireland. Every day that I passed the vine, on the way to and from school, it grew a little longer, until one day it reached the street. Then it was mine. It was my treasure. I held the flowers all day in my hand at school.

I had a lust for plants. The bluebells that grew in the bluebell woods behind our home were not safe from me either. I would travel long distances to find the rare white or pink forms and bring huge bouquets into the house. I put them into jam jars with water. I ate next to them and their perfume, and I read in their company.

One spring morning, I made a very big mistake. The stone terrace in front of my house had an arboretum in it, set out in the mid-1700s. The trees were huge. One squat little tree that was endowed with an armory of thorns decided that it would burst forth into bloom. It was literally covered with flowers. The tree seemed to float up toward the sky, filled with its own pride. I jumped and jumped to secure a piece of branch. With one final fling of my arm I managed to grasp a tip. I walked into the house proudly holding my new treasure on high: a broken branch of hawthorn, *Crataegus monogyna*. I knew its Latin name, too, though I was only seven years old.

I certainly did not expect the hurricane of abuse I received when I entered the house. Simply everybody let out a howl at me. "What do you think you are doing?" The chorus encircled me for the kill. "And what exactly do you think you have in your hand?" I looked down at my new treasure. "Hawthorn," I answered, somewhat scared. Then as if to boost my confidence, I added the condiment to my mistake, *"Crataegus monogyna!"* I should have kept my mouth shut.

My mother took me by the shoulder and pushed me toward the door. She was in flames. She opened the door and deposited me on the doorstep. "Go outside and lose that thing," she ordered. "Don't come back into the house with it in your hand." She glared at me as if I had done something really terrible. "That's hawthorn. It's bad luck to bring it under the roof. It's a magical tree." She slammed the door in my face, as I stood my ground with the flowering branch still firmly grasped in my hot little hand.

That incident was to be my first lesson in magic. And it did not stop me from collecting! What amazed me was the instant reaction of all the adults. It was as if I had let a flock of chickens loose in the house or led a horse into the hall. To a person they were united against my little broken branch of hawthorn with its salad-tasting leaves and chaste white blooms that made my mouth water. I had already made many meals of the red berries the year before, so much so that they dulled my appetite before dinner and I had to pretend to eat. The tree was a nuisance, too. It was difficult to climb. To me it was like Everest, with a huge bole. It was difficult to find a handhold anywhere on the trunk. Now it was forbidden territory, a much more attractive place to be.

In Ireland, the hawthorn has held a magical reputation for thousands of years, stretching to the era of the Druidic priests. The tree was sacred. The tree became a symbol in one of the oldest written languages of Europe, known as Ogham. Ogham script is found on the Ogham stones in Ireland and England, and down to northern Africa. The symbol for hawthorn is simple: half a cross, the cross-bar on the left.

The hawthorn was one of the essential medicines of the Druidic priests, and was commonly used in the treatments of heart disease in both young and old. The haw, or fruit, was eaten either fresh or dried. When fresh, the ones with golden streaks of russeting bear the sweetest berries. The *Crataegus* is a member of the rose or *Rosaceae* family and as such its fruit is technically a pome, bearing five seeds or nutlets.

The haw is considered to be magical by more peoples than the Irish. The Greeks and Romans did also, along with the Chinese and Russians together with many cultures of the Middle East. The North American aboriginal peoples used their haw species in witchcraft. If you wanted to harm someone who had done an injury to you, you used the downy haw,

Crataegus submollis. And if you wanted to reverse
the curse, the dotted haw, *C. punctata*, neutralized the
situation. The interfacing of cultures over time has
probably passed the medicines of one culture on to
another, like the first frosted fruit of the haw being
used by the pioneering farmers of Canada as a trail
food, knowledge that was gathered from aboriginal
experience on this continent.

The haw presents three gifts of medicine to the
world. One is the flower when it is fully open and
presenting its male anthers to the world for
pollination. The second is the modern hypotensive
biochemical the tree manufactures. The third is
the seed crop of nutlets containing caffeine in the
endosperm of the ripe pome or haw.

The beneficial health aspect most available to the
entire household is the scent of the *Crataegus* tree
when it is in full flower. All of the one thousand or
so species of haw across the world carry this chemical
aerosol. In North America, the flower blooms in May.
The entire tree is covered with tiny white flowers in
groupings of about ten per unit, lasting up to two
weeks. Each flower, typically, has five white petals,
like the rose or apple blossom. The female part of

the flower produces a chemical calling card for the insect world to come and pay a visit, released when the white petals are fully open, day after day in the sunshine hours. The aerosol perfume has a clinging action, and can be used as a fixing agent in many over-the-counter perfumes.

The aerosol is a lactone, a scent rising and floating around the inner surface of the male and female parts of the flower. Since the flowers grow in clusters this scent collects until it is quite strong. This is a medicinal aerosol, trapped by the nose and the breathing airways, the most efficient chemical trap of the body. While the aerosol is being sensed by specialized cells, the body goes into action. The salivary gland releases saliva, which pours into the mouth and dissolves the aerosol. This water-soluble medicine travels down into the stomach in a bolus of saliva. Then it goes across the intestinal wall into the body proper.

For some magical and medicinal reason the aerosol keeps going in the circulatory system until it reaches the left ascending coronary artery in the heart. There it stops. The aerosol is finally home and makes its presence felt by opening up the left ascending coronary artery a little wider. This helps the heart to pump more oxygen to itself and into the circulation. The aerosol is a cardiotonic and coronary vasodilator. Its derivatives are used all over the globe by medical practitioners in the treatment of cardiovascular disease.

And this is the magical medicine of the haw, free from the pharmacy of nature.

Wonderful Willows

An old cure to help relieve depression . . .

W hen I was a child in Ireland I loved the milking
cows. My summers were spent on a family
farm called Lisheens. For me the cows and the ritual
of milking by hand were the main attractions. The
huge animals, their gentle ways, their body heat and
their hairy coats filled me with delight. One cow in
particular seemed to return my affection. Her name
was Strawberry. She was a rose-pink colour while
the others were black and white. She was smart and
big-boned. She was the leader of the herd.

After milking every morning, she and the herd
walked the same earthen pathway across one field
called the *Gairdín*, the little garden, and down
another field, the *Droim*, or the back. The pathway
ended at the bottomland of an ancient turf bog
where a small cluster of little willows grew. They were
perched almost horizontally over the flat land using

the tail end of the good soil of the *Droim* to survive. The willows looked so mournful to me. They had nowhere else to go; they stayed in the margins between good and bad soil. But these miserable little trees were like some exotic altar to the cows. Each animal closely followed the other, swinging from side to side with their weight. They jogged down the steep path at an identical slow pace, because of their size and also because cows are no mountain climbers. They ended up fanned around the willows, nosing the leaves with their soft muzzles. The cows would stay there for ages, their feet in the mud, tails switching, arranged like a bouquet around the willows. The hoof patterns, past and present, wet and dry, were a testament to their daily worship.

I often sat on a white rock nearby, watching and waiting. This place at the end of the *Droim* caught the morning sun and was deliciously warm. Strawberry always broke the reverie, the first to move, heading back the way she came for the sweet green grasses and round patches of clovers. The others followed. For the rest of the day the herd made its way, in a black-and-white rosary, back up the *Droim*, lingering at the top of the field before going through the gap in the hedgerow into the *Gairdín*. The line opened a little so the cattle could stroll and graze before they went back to the long, stone, whitewashed milking shed with its smells of sweet hay. Inside, the glittering barley straw on the floor caught the light of the dipping, afternoon sun and seemed to wait for the carillon of songs made by the metal chains used to tie each cow in place.

The unanswered questions of childhood often lead the adult by the hand to find a solution. The willow, *Salix*, is a wonderful genus to me. There are about 300 species. The siblings in this large family simply adore the waterways of the world. See a lake and you will find a willow; find a stream and there will be a willow somewhere nearby. The noblest willow in the world is the weeping willow of China, *Salix babylonica*, a favoured tree in the designs of gardeners everywhere. Close on its heels is the black willow, *S. nigra*, a majestic tree of North America with its habitat ending up in southern Mexico. The black willow with its soft wood is home and haven to many songbirds, butterflies and beneficial pollinating insects up and down the continent.

Across the world in every region the willow
sets the alarm clock for spring. It is one, if not
the first, genus to show signs of growth after the
dormancy of winter. As the days warm, even a little,
the bare tree expands its clutch of male catkins,
which quickly turn yellow. They are loaded down
with rich, nutritional pollen—the first of spring.
It is the most important food source on the planet
for pollinators. Willow pollen feeds honeybees,
wasps, ants, butterflies and the army of winged
pollinators that service the fields of nature.
This pollen contains a key biochemical that is
a springboard to birth. It is called leucine, an
essential amino acid. Without it, proteins cannot
be built, and protein building is necessary to the
life cycle of an insect such as a honeybee or a wasp.
Spring comes early for these creatures. They must
awake and begin work, especially the queen bee.
It is vital that she gets leucine from willow pollen to
begin her long task of laying eggs. Each year she
must produce about 300,000 eggs to make up the
workforce of female honeybees that tend the hive
and fly to feed it with pollen and nectars. This act
of collecting food for the hive cross-pollinates

crops, a minor miracle performed billions of times each year, giving us much of the food for our tables.

Willow trees manufacture some of the most useful medicines known to humankind. One of the most important of these medicines is Aspirin and all of its bio-chemical relatives. Some of these biochemicals track into the damp soil or water around the willow roots. Others stay in the leaves, twigs and stems to shield the tree against disease. And more again are liberated into the air as aerosols. Some react quickly in the tree's vicinity while others float farther away into the ether of a summer's day.

The aboriginal peoples of North America understood the willow. Their medicine men and women used their native willow in the treatment of loneliness and depression. All that is necessary is to sit under the spreading branches of a willow in full canopy and relax your body completely. The tree's aerosols will do the rest.

One question still remains for the child in me: Were the milking cows using the aerosol medicine of the willow on a daily basis, or were they actually in the act of worship?

HONEY LOCUST

A tree that almost sparked a riot . . .

A few years ago I gave a public lecture to a large audience at Harvard University. The back of the hall was set for lunch with tables of white linen and silver. Some kind of buffet was brewing somewhere on campus and was to be brought in at noon. I did not expect the riot that broke out after I gave my talk when some students at the front of the crowd stood up and demanded that I come back to speak to them again. I explained that I was a visitor, I came only by invitation. By the time I was seated at lunch these students had captured an administrator and had brought her to my table. She said, "We will have to have you back."

The subject that had sparked all this excitement was native North American trees. One that captured the students' imagination was the humble honey locust, *Gleditsia triacanthos*, a member of the pea or

Leguminosae family. This tree lives in a wide swath from the Gulf of Mexico up to and beyond the Great Lakes into southern Canada. The long, dangling, sugar-rich pods filled with first-class plant protein once fed the continent's bison herds from the fall into the winter months. The nutritious food made sure that all the female animals in calf stayed healthy and had a good supply of milk to feed their young.

The honey locust is a fodder tree for a farm. In the poorer regions of the United States, the pods are collected for winter feed, like hay. The high protein content of the pods is a boon to a dairy herd's milk production. This protein is, basically, a free supplement.

The leguminous, dry pods can be collected, and the beans or seeds shelled out and prepared like any other dried beans for us to eat. They can also be ground down into nutrient-rich flour or added as a supplement to any other flour to make bread or other baked goods.

The common honey locust was part of a huge geo-engineering experiment in the Dirty Thirties, when year after year of searing sun and drought caused prairie topsoil to flee. Continental topsoil was found as far away as the mid-Atlantic, coating ships in dust and grime. U.S. president Franklin D. Roosevelt ordered the planting of 30,600 kilometres (19,000 miles) of honey locust trees to stabilize the dust bowl lands. The taproot system of the honey locust penetrates the soil to a great depth. Although the roots are devoid of rhizobia bacteria to fix nitrogen, the tree still manages to do it by some unknown mechanism.

The leaves of the honey locust move, shutting down at nightfall. This is unusual. The leaves are doubly compound and about 20 centimetres (8 inches) long, arranged into twenty-eight small oval leaflets ending in a point. When the sun begins to dip in the sky, each leaflet folds into a closed position using the midvein, much like folding a newspaper. This act of shutting down gives the tree its extraordinary ability to survive with very little water, because in the closed position, the stomata are protected from water loss.

The ability of the leaves of the honey locust to fold also gives this tree an ability to survive in dense pollution in industrial cities. It will not only survive, but flourish, generating a canopy that reduces solar exposure and creates shade. The roots are different from many trees, too. They will eke out a living in poor industrial soils, cleaning them and making them richer in carbon and humus. The honey locust and all of its sibling species in South America, Africa, New Zealand, India, China and Japan offer up a cooling effect in the heat race of global warming on the streets of our cities.

Selective breeding experiments at Auburn University in Alabama have shown that the pods of the honey locust can produce as much as 35 percent sugar. In a green economy, this spells alcohol, and alcohol is a very useful fuel. It is possible for a farm to do its own fuel extraction from the sugar-rich pods to run its own machinery, creating a sustainable loop by planting trees and using the fermentation product as fuel and the waste as a nitrogen-rich fertilizer.

The wood of honey locusts is very unusual. It is resistant to the predations of termites. These insects are on the increase with climate change and are moving north as winters grow warmer. The wood is also rot-resistant, making it ideal for window and door making. It takes a very fine polish and can be used as flooring. The timbers can be set in the soil without rotting. This is one reason why so few of these trees exist today. The pioneers used them up. They can be planted again in poor soil and the timber harvested as a green substitute for pressure-treated wood (a multi-billion-dollar industry and growing). Honey locust lumber offers a child-friendly alternative to wood treated with chromated copper arsenate and other toxic preservatives.

Being a member of the pea family, the honey locust produces an extraordinary range of protective medicines. Like all peas, the foliage is delicious to many species of animal, the porcupine being the prime culprit in modern times and the opossum the second best. The tree produces a barbed wire skirt around the trunk to keep them from climbing up into the canopy to feed. The Chinese honey locust, *G. sinensis*, goes one step further with thorns that are branched to protect the foliage. These thorny environments create escape routes and well-guarded resting places for local snake populations.

The bright red thorns of honey locust have the ability to penetrate either human or animal flesh aseptically, meaning they never cause infection. This little trick of the natural world was picked up by the medicine men and women of North America and

China. In ancient times honey locust thorns were the first tools of surgical intervention. In North America, healers collected a series of five identical thorns and inserted them into a wooden handle. This was a trepanning tool for subepidermal surgery used in the treatment of neuralgia and rheumatism.

The use of this instrument was fairly common practice: settlers noticed the series of black dots on the temples of the aboriginal peoples they met, and wrote home to England about them. This simple trephine hid an extraordinary sophistication in medicinal method and understanding. Before use, its tips were plunged into a moistened mixture of black bear gall and charcoal from the native hazel, *Corylus americana*, one that had endogenous fungi in its branches, identified by a bruise-like indentation in the bark. This fungus produces, as its defense mechanism to survive within the hazel, a biochemical box of tricks called taxanes: the mother of all treatments of cancer. The trephine plunged this mixture through the skin and into the surface of the skull, where it travelled into the bloodstream, the charcoal acting as a slow pain-relief mechanism.

Stenocarpine, a local anesthetic, is extracted from honey locust. Probably this biochemical is on call by the tree to increase its nitrogen fix by killing insects that come to pollinate. They fall around the tree, enriching the soil. This tactic is used by a few other trees, such as the white basswood, *Tilia heterophylla*, and insectivorous plants, for instance the pitcher plants, *Sarracenia*, common to Canadian bogs.

The honey locust produces two more active biochemicals: fustin, a potent anti-carcinogenic agent, and fisetin, a biochemical that inhibits aflatoxin, toxins that come into the diet from moulds and bacteria. Some of these come from poor industrial farming practices where mouldy foods are fed to animals and the resulting aflatoxin is still in the meat, milk or eggs. These toxins interact directly with DNA, causing cancers.

The honey locust's spring flowers are fragrant and are a feeding system for the beneficial insects in a city. Its canopy is a gentle one, giving dappled shade, excellent for a city park or garden. Pollution is mopped up and health offered in bounty to the citizens. The sisters of the honey locust can shade the world from Canada to China in places of commerce, bringing the farmer and us back to better days.

Giant Trees

The last of the great living and breathing creatures in the world . . .

The high king of Ireland was called the *Ard-Rí*.
He was the highest king, the king of all the other
smaller kingdoms of Ireland. He unified these kings
in his palace called Tara, where all the learned Celts
came to feast, to listen to the harp, and to expand the
ancient Brehon Laws and codify them.

The last high king was called Brian Boru. He had
a secret. The secret was a forest in County Clare that
was filled with ancient oak trees streaming with ivy,
Hedera helix. The rocks and boulders of this ancient
forest were painted with cloud fern, *Hymenophyllum*.
A singing stream rushed through the length and
breadth of this place that bottled up the sun with its
great, green canopy. Woodcock were flushed with
every step and eaten at every feast.

Of this enormous forest, there remains just one
tree, an oak. The tree has a name. This Irish oak is

called the Brian Boru tree. It is like no other on the planet. The oak stands strong against the hills on a rocky ridge filled with boulders from the last ice age. Its silhouette pictured against the confluence of the skies is like some powerful being. In the early morning the sun climbs like a child into the tree from the horizon of the hills and splashes the green canopy with reflected light that hurts the eyes. From noon onwards the sun hides behind this tree and hangs in the sky, gathering gloom from all the shadows of the past, like a spectre. This oak belongs to the Irish soil. It is the beating heart of Ireland, a green and living organ.

The oak is about a thousand years old. The trunk is colossal and not just one single bole. The branches decided a long time ago to support the tree and are now heavy elbows extending into the fields around, resting on the earth. These elbows have grown adult canopies that add strength to one another, forming a giant green dome of oak leaves and acorns. The roots stray out into the fields and pop up in brown surprise only to dive down into the soil once again.

The horizontal branches hoard soil from bygone ages and spill out with their own territories of ferns. These lanceolate-leaved ferns bend backwards and drip their moisture on the mosses, helping them reproduce and cling to life. The bark of the tree is full of cavities that are like dark caves. There is a special feeling around this tree that seems to drink up everything in the imagination to silence.

A large black Angus bull guards this giant tree. He has an enormous ring in his nose and takes his orders from neither man nor beast. He sleeps in the shade of the tree, day and night, and seems to disappear until he hears a noise. Like a black dog, he challenges everyone, ploughing up the field to defend this giant.

The oak produces a form of black water, which is a medicine of the Celtic Druids. It has taken a thousand years to form from the sheer weight of the trunk and the torque action of the wind on the canopy. The mixture runs like molasses, slowly pouring out of one side of the trunk. This black water would have quercetin in it, but anything else is just a guess. The taste is bittersweet, as would be expected of tannins. This medicine of the Druidic priests has the ability to cure many diseases. It was once considered to be of prime importance in their pharmacopeia of healing.

I walked the walk of the *Ard-Rí*, Brian Boru. I took hundreds of people to the tree to explain its importance to Ireland and to the world. Then I took them on a medicine walk through the Raheen Wood hosted by the Woodland League of Ireland. I spoke about the importance of the common English oak, called *dair* in Irish, and the history it carries into our homes today. I spoke of the sacred woods and groves and demonstrated the extraordinary medicine that once was shared with Europe, and as far as Turkey and northern Africa.

In the evening we returned to the tiny stone chapel Brian Boru had built from large blocks of local stone. The stonemasons had laid down the grey flags in such a way that the resonance of the human voice echoed around and around in this small space. The chapel is called Tuamgraney, and has stood the test of time of a thousand years, like the oak. In this place of ancient prayer, as I spoke more about the healing wisdom and intrinsic value of trees, my voice seemed to carry an edge of the past forward into the future. An Argentinean opera singer sang "Ave Maria" to finish off the evening. We were spellbound together as her notes faded away.

There is a legend in Ireland that the rebuilding of the great forests of the world will begin with the Brian Boru oak and the Raheen Wood. This legend came from a prophecy of Aobhana. She was a Druid, one of the last wise women of Ireland, an advisor to the *Ard-Rí*, Brian Boru.

When the last notes of "Ave Maria" circled the little chapel of Tuamgraney, I felt that every heart there was opened. I became aware of the great power of the human spirit. At that moment I knew for sure that the forest will rise again. I heard it in the song.

Pinene Kids

Pine trees can help kids with learning disorders . . .

Last year I was asked to a birthday party by the River Rats, people who live along the St. Lawrence River that divides the United States from Canada. The River Rats are the offspring of the titans of the manufacturing industries who bought holiday homes to clear the sweat from their unhurried brows during the heat of the summer. Some of them built castles, not the kind that I knew from Ireland, but castles nonetheless, the infection of wealth creeping along on both sides of the river.

The birthday party burst out of the house and down to the rocky banks of the river, overlooking polished wooden skiffs and docks. The sun was frying the grass to cinders and seemed to make the ice sharper in our glasses. The pine trees by the river offered shade, a blessing to everybody who had travelled from afar to be in this place. One was a teacher from

Connecticut. He cut a swath through the crowd directly to me with the homing instinct of a hawk to prey.

We will call him Jack. He headed a school in Connecticut for the mentally challenged boys and girls of our society. They had been put through rigours in the womb. The pregnant moms had either swallowed a bushel of drugs or a lake of alcohol during the nine months their child was in utero, or a gene had unexpectedly malfunctioned. The babies who entered the world were not the perfect creatures their parents had expected. So in due course the parents made their way to Jack's school with a bag of money in one hand and a child in the other, to try to make things better.

Jack's students could walk and run. They looked like ordinary children with the usual whistle of wants. They had the scraped knees and torn clothes of the unruly. Some were beautiful, with the features of angels. All of them suffered from learning disorders. Many were unable to retain instruction, and some had metabolic disorders tied into a lack of logic in thinking. Many had difficulty reading and could not or would not read. Literacy is so vital for modern humans because everything is based on the visuals of letters and numbers.

Year after year, during the heat of the summer, Jack brought his students into the pine woods. They came out calmer, able to focus and to learn. He was getting some serious successes and this had been happening with different groups of students. He could not understand it. The first year he'd seen the results of a walk in the pine woods he thought it was some sort of anomaly that would never happen again.

Connecticut and the eastern seaboard of North America are blessed with pine woods. These pines commonly are the pitch pine, *P. rigida*, now extremely rare in Canada; the eastern white pine, *P. strobus*; the red pine, *P. resinosa*; and the jack pine, *P. banksiana*, made famous by the Group of Seven. There are so many more. Jack took his charges into these pine woods for a walk on a warm summer's day and something very strange happened there. These children felt that the pine trees were communicating with them. All of the kids had the same experience. Each time, kids came out of the pine woods changed. They seemed to settle down. They appeared to be able to focus on learning when they had not been able to do so before their walk. All of them experienced a deep emotional contact with the pine trees. A bonding took place.

The scientific story behind this effect is complicated and wonderful. On a warm, humid, typical summer's day, pine trees liberate a family of aerosols from the rigidly controlled pine needles in the canopy. The variety and amounts of aerosols released are very large. Many of these biochemicals are unusual in their physical chemistry: they can be easily carried about in humid, water-laden air, but they will not dissolve in it, though these pine chemicals will dissolve in chloroforms, ethers and alcohols. All of them are able to penetrate the central nervous system of the human body and the regulatory mechanism of the brain.

Two biochemical aerosols, alpha- and beta-pinene, are released in large amounts into the air on hot summer days. Others arise that may well be just as important. There is an oleoresin or pine resin that is released into the airways around pine trees that also carries the anti-carcinogen limonene, and others. Pines are a source of pine oil and pine tar, all of which are mixtures of active biochemicals capable of interaction with the central nervous system and known to have mild anesthetic properties. In addition, pinosylvin antibiotics are released from the more mature pine trees. This strong antimicrobial is the basis of most of the North American aboriginals' use of pines in their various prescriptive modes.

The aboriginal peoples used pine smoke to prevent sickness of all kinds. A finely ground form of dried pinewood was used as a baby powder and to heal navels. They used shavings from the resin-covered plugs of occluded knots taken from inside the bole of mature pines to treat poison ivy. They were also used as an antibiotic to treat infections.

Pine needle oil extracted from fresh green leaves was used as a medicine in Greek and Roman times. It is currently in use in all the pharmacopeias of Central Europe. Modern multinationals have picked up the message and use it in a number of products such as flavouring, disinfectants, deodorants and solvents.

Returning to Jack's students, maybe all children need nature more than we realize. These children with learning disorders can teach us to look at nature differently. But the fact remains that pine woods benefit all children and have done so for a long time. Maybe we, in science, have something deeper to learn from these pinene kids.

ADDICTION GARDEN

People who suffer from mental illness benefit
deeply from nature . . .

I have felt real fear only twice in my life. It is the kind of fear that attacks your stomach and ties it in knots; the residuals never go away. The memory of the event stays like a stamp in your mind. It reruns without the slightest effort if something steps up to remind you of it once again.

Once when, as a postgraduate student in Ireland, I happened to walk into a small ward in a children's hospital by mistake, a young child was lying in a kind of hammock with her head in a separate one. Her head was enormous. She was born that way, a hydrocephalic. She had an abnormal increase in cerebrospinal fluid within the cranial cavity and expanding cerebral ventricles, all causing an enlargement of the skull, especially the bones of the forehead with a resulting atrophy of the brain. Every move, except that of her eyes, involved immense, rolling, uncontrollable pain. I was frightened of the pastures of pain she still had ahead of her.

Recently I felt the grasp of that fear again. I was invited to an unveiling of a garden that was based on the new thinking of my bioplan concept and a changing regime of treatments at the Centre for Addiction and Mental Health (CAMH). The hospital sits on a 6.9-hectare (17-acre) parcel of land in downtown Toronto. I had to be there by noon. It was a rush for me and I hoped I could make the event in time.

The W. Garfield Weston family was being generous, again, giving to the city they loved through their foundation. The family knew about my research and writing. They invited me through Tree Canada to be the keynote speaker for the media event to announce something new and exciting in the field of mental health.

Jumping out of a taxi, I had difficulty finding the reception area. Nobody I asked knew where I should go. I was in a different world. I had to walk about and find it for myself. I was anxious because I was supposed to be briefed about the protocol of dealing with the media, the various introductions and meeting the Westons.

I am extremely good at getting lost and found
myself walking the various lengths of the ground
floor of the hospital looking for that reception area.
I walked up and down corridors and I passed a great
number of patients. I was mesmerized by what I saw.
I was shocked to see so many young people. The sick
were from every race and corner of the world
imaginable; somehow I did not expect to see so many
men and women, strong or frail. All of these patients,
simply all of them, walked in the same manner with
a form of intense lethargy as if they were in a dream.
They were like zombies, the walking dead.

As I walked along the dull corridors, I became
frightened. I was the oddball, the odd man out. Then
my medical biochemical training began to kick in.
I knew that some were suffering from addictions
and others from true biochemical pathway
malfunctions. There had to be people who were
seriously ill and others who were barely scraping
by in the arena of sanity. All of these people had
different mental diseases, yet were acting in a similar
manner. My fear increased.

I had almost given up finding the reception area
when I noticed the man behind the glass. He had

a cheerful Irish accent and wanted to know how to help. The Irish mafia is alive and well. There is an understanding that all members of the Irish diaspora help one another. He left his desk in the hands of another and went to find my party of people. He came back wearing a broad smile.

Within minutes I was out in the garden, breathing fresh air. I met the donors and the press. The plaque was veiled in a black cloth waiting to be removed and we all crowded around it. My eyes landed on the new wooden benches made of hand-hewn logs that sat under the shade of a grove of maple trees. Here was a healing garden, one in the middle of the city, against the roar of traffic. I began to talk and deliver my ideas about health and the bioplan.

Basically the bioplan takes all that we know about the science of nature and fits it around a problem to find a solution. The patients in CAMH need to be out in the sunshine more than anybody else. They need the vitamin D to boost their immune systems. Trees like the basswood and the catalpa, *Catalpa speciosa*, will bring bees, butterflies and birds into their world again. Others, like the hop hornbeam, *Ostrya virginiana*, will provide calming aerosols. This great restorative garden will continue to be created, planted and enjoyed by the patients. Hands in the soil always heal because nature is the one anchor when all else fails.

THE BIOPLAN

A philosophy to heal the planet . . .

I talk about the bioplan in all my writing. It is the core of my thinking as a scientist. I believe that we are all connected to one another by threads that have already been laid down in nature. To me that means as we stepped out of Africa, the road to discovery began. We are all related to one another in a family that should be blind to race and creed. Our diversity is our blessing and should be the means of our survival, if we are smart enough.

The dignity of humanity extends in grace to the creatures of our world. The whales and other mammals of the oceans breed and nurse their young with a tenderness that we too can feel. The fish monitor their lives by sound. The birds of the air cause the heart to skip with joy when we see the luxury of colour in their feathered breasts. Even the fox that comes into my garden can reflect a form of intelligence in the intensity of his glance that can give me a start and put me in my place.

All of my life I have been a student of nature. Not one single day goes by without my learning something new, something I had never thought of before. The soil is a teacher out there in the vegetable garden. It demands action from me if I am to eat. The trees and orchard conduct their own ceremony of spring with flowers and pollination. I observe and am grateful for what the honeybees and wasps can bring to my plate.

The butterflies weave their generations of cocoons up and down the continent as evidence of their intention to mate and to live. The flash of black and orange from the monarchs as they float overhead is a testament to life itself and to the repeating patterns of unity we drink in from everything that is around us on this planet. It is the unity we find deep within ourselves if we take the time to look.

I begin every day with a poem that clings to my mind for the day. I am grateful for the words of someone else's dream entering my life. Poetry opens the soul and expands the ability to fly with thought and ideas to other places. It is the closest I will get to my core, to my own science, on a daily basis.

It takes a certain amount of moral courage to stand within the breakers of the ocean of our own discontent and to hang on to the ideas of the destiny of humankind. We are a people of privilege; we know right from wrong. That knowledge is not outside of us, it is within. We must look inside to find the solutions to put nature right, to mend the pieces, to put it back together again. We must all do it together.

We can use my idea of the bioplan to patch the places that need mending if all of us, each one of us, can pay attention to our own backyard. We will succeed because piece by piece the puzzle will go back to the clear view of nature that our own human family once had.

Here is how I define my term, bioplan, which I first described in my book, *A Garden for Life*: "the bioplan is a blueprint for all connectivity of life in nature. It is the fragile web that keeps each creature in balance with its neighbour. It is predator and prey. It is the victor and victim in a vast cycle of elemental life that is almost beyond our comprehension. It is the quantum mechanic of the green chloroplast without which we would all die. It is the trichoma on the underside of deciduous trees harbouring parasites for aphids. It is the ultraviolet traffic light signalling system in flowers used by the insect world. It is the terpene aerosol SOS produced by plants in response to invasive damage. It is the toxin trick offered by plants for the protection of butterflies. It is the mantle of man, in his life and in his death, a divine contract, to all who share this planet."

The bioplan tells us that one cannot remove the forests of Borneo and Sumatra and expect the orangutans to live. Nor can one remove the temperate rainforests of the west coast of Canada and see salmon coming back to the rivers. Nor can we allow the 200,000 hectares (about 500,000 acres) of mature forest to be removed from Nova Scotia to provide wood pellets for Boston, or the boreal forest for oil extraction. Some foundations of nature have to remain. We must all see to this, beginning at our own doorstep. The cities must do their piece, also, by planting urban forests of the native trees that once stood in place of concrete. Both can go together, for the benefit of everybody.

Real health is found through nature. It simply does not make any sense to have a quadruple bypass and to

go out into your garden a month later to rest and
relax, only to be stung by a mosquito carrying West
Nile virus or encephalitis because the bats and birds
disappeared due to starvation or disease because the
trees were cut down. This is true for the Amazon and
now for most of the rest of the world including our
great cities of Montreal, Ottawa, Toronto, Calgary,
Edmonton, Vancouver . . . We should not have to worry
about a visit to the surgeon for a bone transplant that
carries a prion from a cadaver that succumbed to
Jakob-Creutzfeldt Disease. Doctors can treat disease,
but there is no remedy for stupidity. It is stupid to pull
nature apart and expect people to be healthy.

Then there is the general health of the planet to be
considered. Today the great tropical forests with all
of their antiviral medicines are being ripped out of
the islands of southeast Asia. Today the seascape
of our great oceans is being destroyed by dragnets
as our governments stand and watch. Their silence
is deafening. Their lobby is invisible.

Tomorrow, you will plant a tree. Then you and your
friends will plant more. Together we can do it. We can
hold hands across the planet and repair the damage
done in the past five hundred years. Hand by hand we

will make a daisy chain of people willing to improve our lot and that of all others. We will make a difference to nature, one by one and tree by tree. The roots will grow to anchor the forest back to the power of the sun and rekindle the life we all so richly deserve. Again. For all the tomorrows to come.

Trees in the Millennium Project . . .

1. The bur oak, *Quercus macrocarpa*. This edible oak is the best tree to aid in carbon sequestration in the eastern portion of North America. The demand for oak is increasing in the wine trade.

2. The Thomas walnut, *Juglans nigra* 'Thomasii.' A perennially bearing tree of very sweet walnuts. The bole is extremely straight in this handsome tree.

3. The Carrigliath black walnut, *J. n.* 'Carrigliath.' An anti-famine tree whose nuts hold a sweet taste on the palate like the pecan. This tree was selected from nut trials here in the garden.*

4. The Burwell black walnut, *J. n.* 'Burwell.' A very hardy northern walnut. It is an excellent forest tree with edible nuts.*

5. The butternut, *J. cinerea* 'Batesii,' named for Mr. Meryl Bates, a farmer, who collected the original trees from the virgin forest of Ontario over a hundred years ago.

The nutmeats are excellent for winter storage and kitchen use.*

6. The Canadian shagbark hickory, *Carya ovata* 'Carrigliath,' is a product of seed selection and ongoing field trials in the garden. The nutmeats hold a creamy taste and are excellent for nut milks, creams and curds. They are high in essential fatty acids, oleic and linoleic.*

7. The hackberry, also known as the sugarberry, *Celtis occidentalis*. This is a feeding tree for wildlife. It also holds commercial applications for rope making.

8. The Canadian red oak, *Quercus rubra*, is an ornamental tree for its wonderful foliage and acorn crop for wildlife.

9. The Canadian plum, *Prunus nigra*, this small native tree feeds all kinds of beneficial predatory species and pollinating insects in the garden.

10. The wild sweet crabapple, *Malus coronaria*, a native apple of Canada with extra sweetly scented spring bloom and small apples. It is a pollinating tree beloved by bluebirds and fall warblers.

11. The witch hazel, *Hamamelis virginiana*, a favourite tree of the Iroquois nation, with medicinal properties.

12. The pawpaw tree, *Asimina triloba*, could be an important new health food for the twenty-first century worldwide.

13. The nannyberry, *Viburnum lentago*, with edible fruit that tastes like dates. It is much beloved by larger birds like grouse and turkeys.

14. The silky dogwood, *Cornus amomum*, also called kinnikinnik in Algonquian. It was mixed with tobacco and smoked. This is a butterfly and wildlife tree.

15. The orchid tree, *Catalpa speciosa* 'Carrigliath.' This tree is also called the Indian bean tree. A magnificent North American native grown from hand-selected seeds and field-trialed for hardiness in the garden. It attracts butterflies with its flowers and is a feeding tree for beneficial insects with extra floral nectary.*

16. The common buttonbush, *Cephalanthus occidentalis*, the rare and famous butterfly-feeding tree for the continent of North America.

17. The sour cherry, *Prunus cerasus* var. *austera*, a yearly cropper and a must for every kitchen garden. The pies are heavenly.

18. A standard Russian apple, the Duchess of Oldenburg apple, an early cropping apple that is frost-resistant with fragrant sweet apples for cooking or eating.

19. The standard Russian pear, *Pyrus ussuriensis*, for its early spring blossom, beauty and crop of small pears for wildlife.

20. The wafer ash, *Ptelea trifoliata*. The most fragrant native tree on the continent, smelling of hyacinths. It is a medicinal tree of the orange family.

21. The cucumber tree, *Magnolia acuminata*, is a spring beauty with its grey blossoms and cucumbers in the fall that feed wildlife. It is a beloved tree of the Huron nation for the magical face masks made from its wood.

22. The tulip tree, *Liriodendron tulipifera*, a spectacular tree carrying huge yellow tulips smelling of melon and splashed with streaks of red. It, too, is a medicinal tree.

Numbers 20, 21 and 22 were reserved for experienced gardeners only. Quality substitutes for nut trees can be obtained from specialty nurseries like the following:

Grimo Nut Nursery
979 Lakeshore Road
R.R. 3, Niagara-on-the-Lake
Ontario L0S 1J0
Phone: 905-934-6887
www.grimonut.com

Rhora's Nut Farm and Nursery
33083 Wills Road
R.R. 1, Wainfleet
Ontario L0S 1V0
Phone: 905-899-3508
www.nuttrees.com

* These were selected varieties developed in my garden, Carrigliath. *Juglans nigra*, *Juglans cinerea*, *Carya ovata* and *Catalpa speciosa* trees are available in several outstanding varieties from a number of different suppliers.

References

Anonymous. "Log Tale. Deforestation in Sarawak"
The Economist, November 3, 2012,75.
——. "Fish and Chips." *The Economist,* May 29, 2010, 81.
Editorial. "A man of vision." *Ottawa Citizen,* August 6,
2011, B6.
Béliveau, Richard, and Denis Gingras. *Foods That Fight
Cancer: Preventing Cancer Through Diet.* Toronto:
McClelland and Stewart, 2006.
Beresford-Kroeger, Diana. *Arboretum America: A Philosophy
of the Forest.* Ann Arbor: University of Michigan
Press, 2003.
——. *Arboretum Borealis: A Lifeline of the Planet.* Ann Arbor:
University of Michigan Press, 2010.
——. *A Garden for Life.* Ann Arbor: University of Michigan
Press, 2004.
——. *The Global Forest.* New York: Viking, 2010.
——. "King of the Forest." *Nature Canada,* spring 2000, 16–19.
Buettner, Dan. "The Island Where People Forget to Die."
The New York Times, October 28, 2012.

Byers, Shirley. "How plants communicate with each other and with other life forms." *Small Farm Canada*, September/October, 2012, 7.

Collingwood, G.H., and Warren Bush. *Knowing Your Trees*. Washington, D.C.: American Forestry Association, 1974.

Coombes, Allen J. *The Book of Leaves*. Chicago: University of Chicago Press, 2010.

Crofton, Kerry. *Wireless Radiation Rescue*. Global Well-being Books, 2010.

Densmore, F. *Indian Use of Wild Plants for Crafts, Food, Medicine and Charms*. Oksweken: Iroqrafts, 1993.

Friedman, Joseph, Sarah Kraus, Yirmi Hauptman, Yoni Schiff and Rony Seger. "Mechanism of short-term ERK activation by electromagnetic fields at mobile phone frequencies." *Biochemical Journal,* Vol. 405, 2007, 559–568.

Fulda, S. *et al*. "Betulinic acid: a new cytotoxic agent against malignant brain tumour cells." *International Journal of Cancer*, 1999, 435–441.

Fullbright, Dennis W. *A Guide to Nut Tree Culture in North America*. Vol 1. East Lansing: Northern Nut Growers Association, 2003.

Herrick, James W. *Iroquois Medical Botany*. Syracuse: Syracuse University Press, 1995.

Hillier, Harold. *The Hillier Manual of Trees and Shrubs*. Newton Abbot: David and Charles Redwood, 1992.

Lee, Robert Edward. *Phycology.* 2ⁿᵈ ed. Cambridge:
    Cambridge University Press, 1995.

Lewis, Walter H., and Memory P.F. Elvin-Lewis. *Medical
    Botany: Plants Affecting Human Health.* Hoboken, N.J.:
    John Wiley and Sons, 2003.

Liberty Hyde Bailey Hortorium. *Hortus Third: A Concise
    Dictionary of Plants Cultivated in the United States and
    Canada.* New York: Macmillan, 1976.

Marles, Robin J., Christine Clavelle, Leslie Monteleone,
    Matalie Tays, and Donna Burns. *Aboriginal Plant Use in
    Canada's Northwest Boreal Forest.* Vancouver: University
    of British Columbia Press, 2000.

Milius, Susan. "How elephants call long-distance." *Science
    News,* September 8, 2012, 11.

Myers, Norman. *Gaia: An Atlas of Planet Management.*
    New York: Doubleday, 1984.

O'Neil, Mary Adele J. *The Merck Index: An Encyclopedia of
    Chemicals, Drugs, and Biologicals.* 14ᵗʰ ed. Whitehouse
    Station, N.J.: Merck, 2006.

Packenham, Thomas. *In Search of Remarkable Trees:
    On Safari in Southern Africa.* New York: Walker, 2007.

Pishu, E., *et al.* "Discovery of betulinic acid as a selective
    inhibitor of human melanoma that functions by
    induction apoptosis. *Nature—Medicine,* 1995,
    1046-1051.

Purseglove, J.W. *Tropical Crops: Dicotyledons.* 2 vols.
    New York: John Wiley and Sons, 1968.

———. *Tropical Crops: Monocotyledons*. Harlow: Longman Group Limited, 1972.

Rackham, Oliver. *The Illustrated History of the Countryside*. London: George Weidenfeld and Nicholson, 1994.

Raloff, Janet. "Chemicals linked to kids' lower IQs." *Science News,* May 21, 2011, 15.

———. "Nanopollutants pose crop risks." *Science News*, October 6, 2012, 18.

———. "Extreme heat rising worldwide." *Science News*, September 8, 2012, 10.

———. "Elevated carbon dioxide may impair reasoning." *Science News* (web edition), October 16, 2012.

———. "Night lights may foster cancer." *Science News*, January 19, 2008, 45.

Rix, Martyn, and Roger Phillips. *The Bulb Book*. London: Pan Books, 1981.

Saunders, Laura. "Gene connects lack of shut-eye with diabetes." *Science News*, January 3, 2009, 5–6.

Schopmeyer, C.S. *Seeds of Woody Plants in the United States*. Washington, D.C.: Forest Service, U.S. Department of Agriculture, 1974.

Spinella, Marcello. *The Psychopharmacology of Herbal Medicine*. Cambridge, MA: MIT Press, 2001.

Stuart, Malcolm. *The Encyclopedia of Herbs and Herbalism*. London: Orbix, 1979.

Sun, I.C., H.K. Woong, Y. Kashiwada, J.K. Shen, L.M. Cosentino, C.H. Chea, L.M. Yang, and K.H. Lee.

"Anti-AIDS agents." *Journal of Medical Chemistry*, 1998, 4648–4657.

Turner, Nancy V. *Plants of Haida Gwaii*. Winlaw, B.C.: SONO NIS Press, 2010.

Williams, Michael. *Deforesting the Earth, from Prehistory to Global Crisis, An Abridgement*. Chicago: University of Chicago Press, 2006.

World Health Organization Global Health Observatory. "Urban population" growth: http://www.who.int/gho/urban_health/situation_trends/urban_population_growth_text/en/index.html. Accessed 2013-03-12.

Acknowledgements

These people come into the kingdom of my writing and
I am so glad that they are there. Christian, my husband,
is my support and administrative expert. Nancy Wortman
returns my manuscripts to me with perfection. Lynn,
her husband, keeps a techno eye on the process. Erika
Beresford-Kroeger, my daughter, and her partner, Terence
Moore, and Mary Kate Laphen helped with research. As
editor, Anne Collins matched her challenging scrawl with
mine. Amanda Lewis gave the Irish touch. Stuart Bernstein
played the agent's tune from New York, with kind advice
and encouragement. Thank you, to all of you, again.

DIANA BERESFORD-KROEGER, a botanist, medical biochemist and self-defined "renegade scientist," brings together ethnobotany, biochemistry, horticulture, spirituality and alternative medicine to reveal a path toward better stewardship of the natural world. In 2010, Beresford-Kroeger was inducted as a Wings Worldquest Fellow. The *Utne Reader* named her one of their Visionaries for 2011. In the same year she was elected as a fellow of the Royal Canadian Geographical Society. She lives in Ontario with her husband, Christian H. Kroeger, surrounded by her research garden, Carrigliath, filled with rare and endangered species.

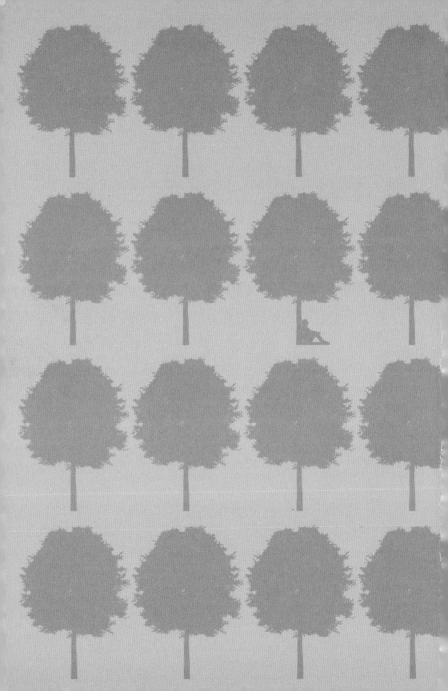